Observations on the prognostic in acute diseases. By Charles Le Roy, M.D. F.R.S. ... Translated from the French. With notes.

Charles Le Roy

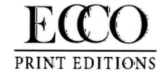

ECCO
PRINT EDITIONS

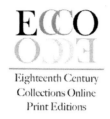

Gale ECCO Print Editions

Relive history with *Eighteenth Century Collections Online*, now available in print for the independent historian and collector. This series includes the most significant English-language and foreign-language works printed in Great Britain during the eighteenth century, and is organized in seven different subject areas including literature and language; medicine, science, and technology; and religion and philosophy. The collection also includes thousands of important works from the Americas.

The eighteenth century has been called "The Age of Enlightenment." It was a period of rapid advance in print culture and publishing, in world exploration, and in the rapid growth of science and technology – all of which had a profound impact on the political and cultural landscape. At the end of the century the American Revolution, French Revolution and Industrial Revolution, perhaps three of the most significant events in modern history, set in motion developments that eventually dominated world political, economic, and social life.

In a groundbreaking effort, Gale initiated a revolution of its own: digitization of epic proportions to preserve these invaluable works in the largest online archive of its kind. Contributions from major world libraries constitute over 175,000 original printed works. Scanned images of the actual pages, rather than transcriptions, recreate the works *as they first appeared.*

Now for the first time, these high-quality digital scans of original works are available via print-on-demand, making them readily accessible to libraries, students, independent scholars, and readers of all ages.

For our initial release we have created seven robust collections to form one the world's most comprehensive catalogs of 18th century works.

Initial Gale ECCO Print Editions collections include:

History and Geography
Rich in titles on English life and social history, this collection spans the world as it was known to eighteenth-century historians and explorers. Titles include a wealth of travel accounts and diaries, histories of nations from throughout the world, and maps and charts of a world that was still being discovered. Students of the War of American Independence will find fascinating accounts from the British side of conflict.

Social Science

Delve into what it was like to live during the eighteenth century by reading the first-hand accounts of everyday people, including city dwellers and farmers, businessmen and bankers, artisans and merchants, artists and their patrons, politicians and their constituents. Original texts make the American, French, and Industrial revolutions vividly contemporary.

Medicine, Science and Technology

Medical theory and practice of the 1700s developed rapidly, as is evidenced by the extensive collection, which includes descriptions of diseases, their conditions, and treatments. Books on science and technology, agriculture, military technology, natural philosophy, even cookbooks, are all contained here.

Literature and Language

Western literary study flows out of eighteenth-century works by Alexander Pope, Daniel Defoe, Henry Fielding, Frances Burney, Denis Diderot, Johann Gottfried Herder, Johann Wolfgang von Goethe, and others. Experience the birth of the modern novel, or compare the development of language using dictionaries and grammar discourses.

Religion and Philosophy

The Age of Enlightenment profoundly enriched religious and philosophical understanding and continues to influence present-day thinking. Works collected here include masterpieces by David Hume, Immanuel Kant, and Jean-Jacques Rousseau, as well as religious sermons and moral debates on the issues of the day, such as the slave trade. The Age of Reason saw conflict between Protestantism and Catholicism transformed into one between faith and logic -- a debate that continues in the twenty-first century.

Law and Reference

This collection reveals the history of English common law and Empire law in a vastly changing world of British expansion. Dominating the legal field is the *Commentaries of the Law of England* by Sir William Blackstone, which first appeared in 1765. Reference works such as almanacs and catalogues continue to educate us by revealing the day-to-day workings of society.

Fine Arts

The eighteenth-century fascination with Greek and Roman antiquity followed the systematic excavation of the ruins at Pompeii and Herculaneum in southern Italy; and after 1750 a neoclassical style dominated all artistic fields. The titles here trace developments in mostly English-language works on painting, sculpture, architecture, music, theater, and other disciplines. Instructional works on musical instruments, catalogs of art objects, comic operas, and more are also included.

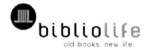

The BiblioLife Network

This project was made possible in part by the BiblioLife Network (BLN), a project aimed at addressing some of the huge challenges facing book preservationists around the world. The BLN includes libraries, library networks, archives, subject matter experts, online communities and library service providers. We believe every book ever published should be available as a high-quality print reproduction; printed on-demand anywhere in the world. This insures the ongoing accessibility of the content and helps generate sustainable revenue for the libraries and organizations that work to preserve these important materials.

The following book is in the "public domain" and represents an authentic reproduction of the text as printed by the original publisher. While we have attempted to accurately maintain the integrity of the original work, there are sometimes problems with the original work or the micro-film from which the books were digitized. This can result in minor errors in reproduction. Possible imperfections include missing and blurred pages, poor pictures, markings and other reproduction issues beyond our control. Because this work is culturally important, we have made it available as part of our commitment to protecting, preserving, and promoting the world's literature.

GUIDE TO FOLD-OUTS MAPS and OVERSIZED IMAGES

The book you are reading was digitized from microfilm captured over the past thirty to forty years. Years after the creation of the original microfilm, the book was converted to digital files and made available in an online database.

In an online database, page images do not need to conform to the size restrictions found in a printed book. When converting these images back into a printed bound book, the page sizes are standardized in ways that maintain the detail of the original. For large images, such as fold-out maps, the original page image is split into two or more pages

Guidelines used to determine how to split the page image follows:

• Some images are split vertically; large images require vertical and horizontal splits.
• For horizontal splits, the content is split left to right.
• For vertical splits, the content is split from top to bottom.
• For both vertical and horizontal splits, the image is processed from top left to bottom right.

OBSERVATIONS

ON THE

PROGNOSTIC

IN

ACUTE DISEASES.

BY

CHARLES LE ROY, M.D. FR.S.

REGIUS PROFESSOR OF PHYSIC, IN THE UNIVERSITY OF
MONTPELLIER, AND MEMBER OF THE ROYAL
SOCIETY OF PHYSICIANS, AT PARIS, &c.

TRANSLATED FROM THE FRENCH.

WITH

NOTES.

LONDON,

Printed for G. WILKIE, No. 71, St. Paul's Church-Yard.

MDCCLXXXII.

PREFACE.

THE great end of physic being
to diſtinguiſh, and to cure
diſeaſes; ſuch publications, as are
the reſult of long experience, and a
judicious and attentive obſervation,
cannot be too generally read. The
art of Prognoſticating in physic, has
always been conſidered as a very eſ-
ſential proof of a phyſician's knowledge; and his abilities in his pro-
feſſion are very often meaſured by his

ſkill

ſkill in this department: nor is this altogether without reaſon, becauſe no man can foreſee what is likely to happen in an Acute Diſeaſe, who is not thoroughly acquainted with its nature, and, at the ſame time, able to diſtinguiſh, with accuracy, all the ſigns it affords, and then, after tracing each of theſe, to its moſt probable cauſe, to weigh theſe cauſes with preciſion, and compare them with each other, and with the natural powers of the patient. The Prognoſtic has, therefore, an intimate affinity with the Diagnoſtic, and this knowledge evidently requires an extenſive acquaintance with books and nature. A phyſician, who excels in this art, muſt have ſtudied diſeaſes, both in his cloſet, and at the bed-ſide of the ſick. He muſt, likewiſe,

wife, poffefs a clear, fteady, and penetrating judgement, which fuffers
no fymptom, not even the moft
minute one, to efcape him, and
which knows how to give to each
fymptom its juft value. Thefe are
qualities, which every practitioner
does not poffefs, and even they who
do, will probably not be difpleafed
to have an ufeful compendium, which
may facilitate their ftudies in this
way. Every man, who aims at
practifing with reputation, will naturally wifh to improve his knowledge of the Prognoftics, becaufe,
without fuch a knowledge, he will
be expofed to endlefs errors, and
mortifications. He will, perhaps,
pronounce, that a patient is out of
danger, who fhall die in the night;
or, that another is dying, when nature

ture is really bringing about some salutary change. One of the first questions, that a patient, or his friends, put to a physician, is, " *Do you think there is danger ?*" or, " *Do you give us any hopes ?*" and how will that man be esteemed, whose Prognostic is every day contradicted by the event, and who flatters the hopes of a family, when a father, or a husband, or a daughter, are at the brink of inevitable death; or who brings grief and sorrow to the bed-side, when the patient is out of danger. Yet these are no imaginary cases, but facts, which every day occur, to the disgrace, not of physic, but to those who stile themselves physicians.

The

The ancients, who ftudied nature in herfelf, were extremely attentive to the figns of difeafes, and, of courfe, were well fkilled in the art of Prognofticating. Semeiology, or the doctrine of figns, was, confeffedly, the beft and moft ufeful part of the medical knowledge of the ancients. All experienced phyficians, have ftudied the Prognoftics in the writings of Hippocrates, but even the moft judicious admirers of that divine old man, are obliged to confefs, that many of his Prognoftics are defective. Some of them are evidently contrary to experience. Others are delivered in a general manner, altho' applicable only to particular cafes. Many of his Prognoftics are delivered as certain, which have a claim only to probability. We fhall very often find

find him giving some particular signs as the forerunners of death, but which commonly announce, only more or less danger. In short, many of his Prognostics, (either through the obscurity of the stile, or from the diseases, to which they relate, not being sufficiently known) are altogether unintelligible, and have even been the subject of controversy. There was, therefore, no other way to rectify these mistakes, and establish the science of Prognostics on a clear and coherent basis, than by attending carefully to nature, and comparing the signs and events of diseases, with what we find delivered by Hippocrates, and other good writers; and with what might have occurred to the observer himself, in the course of his practice. A work,

judiciously

judiciously executed on such a plan, was a desideratum in physic.

Prosper Alpini's seven books, *De presagienda vita et morte*, have long been in great repute with physicians. Whoever reads them, sees, at once, all the doctrine of the ancients on this subject, but he copied from them indiscriminately, without distinguishing between truth and error.

The author of the following work, informs us, in his preface, that his first care was to divest himself of all superstitious veneration for the writings of Hippocrates; that he has carefully compared the Prognostics of Hippocrates with his own observations; adopting such as were conformable to truth; and correcting

b or

or rejecting, such as were defective or erroneous; that he has had in his eye the best writings on this subject; and has availed himself of such lights, as the frequent dissection of morbid bodies, has occasionally thrown on the subject.

" In the almost infinite number
" of signs," says the ingenious author, " which Acute Diseases afford
" us, there are only some few that
" are peculiar to any one of these
" diseases. All the others are com-
" mon to them, and have, therefore,
" the same Prognostic signification,
" whether it be in inflammation of
" the breast, or in continued fevers,
" or small-pox, &c. Hence the
" utility of treating the Prognos-
" tic in these diseases, in a gene-
" ral

" general way, and with all the
" extent it merits; and which could
" not be done with each of these
" diseases, separately, without fall-
" ing into continual repetitions.
" Hippocrates was aware of the
" great utility of such a plan, which
" he has accordingly adopted, in his
" book, *De Prænotionibus*, which
" is, perhaps, the best, or at least,
" the most exact of all his writings.
" The present work is formed on the
" same plan. It is, particularly, in-
" tended for young physicians. I
" hope it may contribute, to facili-
" tate their progress in the art of
" Prognostics, and likewise lead
" them to relish and understand the
" writings of Hippocrates, and to
" distinguish the little taste and dif-
" cernment of the greater number of
" his commentators. In short, I

" flatter

" flatter myſelf, that it will tend to
" remove ſome of the difficulties
" which muſt neceſſarily be ſur-
" mounted, before we can make
" any proficiency in this intereſting
" branch of phyſic.

" Confining myſelf to the ſimple
" narration of facts, my great aim has
" been, to be conciſe, without being
" obſcure. I have very ſeldom ſpo-
" ken of any Prognoſtics, that I have
" not ſeen confirmed in my own
" practice ; and if I have ſometimes
" deviated from the rule, I had laid
" down in this reſpect, it has only
" been for a ſmall number of Prog-
" noſtics, the truth of which ſeem-
" ed to be confirmed, by ſo many ob-
" ſervations, and by writers of ſuch
" weight, that it would have been
" exceeding

" exceeding the bounds of a prudent
" referve, not to have inferted them
" in this work.

" The reader will, very often, find
" a confiderable difference between
" the Prognoftics of Hippocrates,
" and thofe of this work, which re-
" fer to him. In fome, I fhall be
" found giving a literal tranflation
" of him, and in others, faying more
" than he fays. The judicious rea-
" der, will eafily conceive my reafons
" for fo doing. Whenever the affer-
" tions of Hippocrates, are clear, and
" evidently conformable to experi-
" ence, I content myfelf, with giving
" his expreffions; but whenever he is
" too concife, or obfcure, or contra-
" dictory to experience, I have at-
" tempted to rectify the defect.

" In a work of this fort, only by
" much the fmaller number of Prog-
" noftics, can be delivered as certain-
" ties : the reft will vary in their de-
" grees of probability. It has, there-
" fore, been my aim, to adapt my ex-
" preffions to the degree of probabi-
" lity, which feemed to belong to
" each Prognoftic."

To this account of the work, the
Editor has only to add, that in his
tranflation, he has endeavoured to
adhere clofely to the fenfe, and expreffions, of the original ; and he
flatters himfelf, that the notes, he
has occafionally added, will, in fome
meafure, improve the utility of the
performance.

A D V E R-

ADVERTISEMENT.

THE reader will meet with different kinds of references in the courfe of this work, The Roman numbers included in a parenthefis, (§ cccl.) refer to different paragraphs of the work. The Arabic numbers, preceded by an afterifm. (* 14.) refer to the notes at the end of the work ; and the numbers preceded by thefe three letters, *Hip.* refer to the Prognoftics of Hippocrates, on Acute Difeafes, which are collected together at page 197, *et feq.* At the end of each of thefe Prognoftics, care has been taken to indicate, from what part of the writings of Hippocrates they have been collected. Zuinger's edition * has been followed, in the numbers which diftinguifh the paragraphs, taken from the *Prænotiones,* and *Prænot. Coac.*

All the notes, at the bottom of a page, are by the editor.

---

* *Magni Hippocrates coi opufcula aphoriftica, &c.* Bafilæ, 1748.

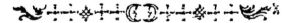

OF THE
PROGNOSTIC
IN
ACUTE DISEASES.

TO arrange in due order in our memory the figns which indicate the Prognoftic in acute difeafes, and to enable us to obferve them advantageoufly at the bed-fide of the fick; we muft neceffarily confider by what feries of effects thefe difeafes become dangerous, and even mortal; and in what way they are to be cured. It is the total ceffation of the circulation of the blood that conftitutes death. This is the boundary to which all mortal difeafes tend. Their effect is therefore gradually to weaken this function, till the moment in which it is altogether extinguifhed. This is their ultimate effect. It is indeed an internal

B   one,

one, and beyond the reach of our fenfes; but it is acceffible by many fecondary and fenfible effects, which being derived from it, become fo many figns of this internal effect of the difeafe. Thefe figns of a languid and nearly extinguifhed circulation, are chiefly an exceffive weaknefs of the whole body, pulfe, and countenance, a great change in the phyfiognomy, and coldnefs of the extremities; the ends of the fingers and toes, and even fome parts of the face, have, at the fame time, a livid afpect. Daily experience proves the connexion of the fecondary and fenfible effects, with the languor of the circulation which occafions them, and which they, in their turn, ferve to indicate. The greater or lefs degree of fagacity in the phyfician, in forefeeing the approaching death of his patient, depends therefore on his ability to obferve and underftand thefe figns. It will depend, likewife, on the other figns which the difeafe may have prefented, or continues to prefent; and which weaken or confirm the Prognoftic of an inevitable and fpeedy death,

death, according as they are found to indicate, either that the viscera are in a
found state, or that some one among them
is grievously affected.

It does not indeed often happen, that
the gradual weakening, and the total cessation of the circulation, are the immediate effect of the disease. Its first attacks
are usually on some particular viscus,
which becoming mortally affected, does,
in its turn put a total stop to the circulation. At the beginning of many acute
diseases which become mortal, the vital
powers seem to be increased, instead
of being diminished. When they become so far weakened, as to give room to
foresee the approach of death, this event
seems almost constantly to be clearly determined by the influence of the disease
on some particular viscus, by the alarming and irremediable affection it has occasioned in it. Without speaking of the
peripneumony, of the hepatitis, and
other diseases of the same class, where the
inflammation of the particular viscus is

evident

evident from the very firſt attack : it is a familiar faƈt, that the acute fevers, which have been named idiopathic ones; and likewiſe, eruptive fevers, as the ſmall pox and meaſles, become mortal, only ſo often as ſome internal part, durıng their courſe, becomes irremediably injured. Sometimes we ſee this fatal influence determined to the brain or its meninges; ſometimes to the lungs or the pleura; and ſometimes to one or other of the abdominal viſcera.

ALTHOUGH, from their particular nature, peſtilential and malignant fevers would ſeem immediately to weaken the circulatory organs and vital powers; yet they prove mortal in the ſame manner. It indeed ſometimes happens in the plague, that the circulation of the blood, is, as it were, ſuffocated, and that the patient dies in the very horripilatio that marks the attack of the diſeaſe. A ſyncope happening in the courſe of a peſtilential or malignant fever, is ſometimes ſufficient to occaſion the death of the patient, which

ſeems

feems then to be determined folely by the impreffion of the difeafe on the organs of circulation: but thefe events are rare. The ufual progrefs of thefe difeafes, when they become mortal, is to excite, either at their beginning or during their courfe, an irremediable affection of fome particular vifcus. This appears from the fucceffive chain of fymptoms in thefe difeafes when they terminate in death. In fome it is a phrenitic delirium, in others a comatofe affection; now and then it is epileptic convulfions that characterize the melancholy influence of the difeafe on the brain or its meninges. A very painful ftitch in the fide, together with a difficulty of breathing, will announce its influence on the lungs or the pleura. An exceffive elevation of the lower belly, or a fenfible and painful tumefaction of any particular part of that cavity, will likewife occafionally point out the effects of the difeafe to be on fome one or more of the abdominal vifcera.

THE

THE diffections of fubjects who have died of Acute Difeafes, whether idiopathic or fymptomatic, inflammatory or malignant, confirm what I have now advanced on the internal caufes of the fymptoms they difclofe. Thefe diffections prove the connexion of thefe fymptoms with the internal affections they indicate. They prove, at the fame time, that a man rarely falls a victim to an Acute Difeafe, without there appearing on diffection, evident marks of the difeafe having more or lefs affected certain vifcera, either by inflammation or abfcefs, or gangrene, or purulent, or gangrenous fpots; or fometimes, by producing an exudation or extravafation into fome one of the three cavities.

OUR books abound with obfervations in confirmation of this doctrine. It is indeed a truth that is adopted by all experienced phyficians who attend carefully to difeafes. It is on this that their enquiries at each vifit are founded, and by which they aim at difcovering how much

much any of the viscera are disturbed or injured. It is a common language with practitioners in acute fevers, to say, " *The viscera or the cavities are free;*" or, that " *the disease threatens to attack, or has attacked the head, the breast, or the lower belly;*" or, that " *it affects such and such viscera, that this affection is trifling, or that it is alarming.*" All these expressions mark at once the degree of hope or fear they conceive from the symptoms of the disease, to be proportioned to the state of the viscera, or to the injury with which one or more of them seem to be menaced.

Such is therefore the ordinary progress of diseases when they become mortal. They begin by injuring some particular viscus, and this affection, when in a certain degree, gradually weakens the power of the circulation, and at length occasions its total cessation. This likewise is the usual progress of deep wounds, or of the inflammation and gangrene of external parts. Whenever the operation for the

stone

ftone is followed by death, this event is
to be attributed to the inflammation that
takes place in the bladder and parts around
it. The mortal difeafe that fometimes
follows fuch an operation, begins at firft
with acute fever, together with a gliftening, pain, and extreme fenfibility in the
hypograftic region, which denotes the inflammation of the parts I have mentioned;
and this inflammation, when arrived at
a certain degree, will occafion the great
diminution of the pulfe, and all the other
ufual forerunners of a fpeedy and inevitable death. If the inflammation of any
tendinous part, or a compound fracture, or
an amputation, are fucceeded by death;
we conftantly obferve in the courfe of
either of thefe difeafes, that independent of the fever, either phrenitic delirium, or tetanos, or comatofe affection,
or great difficulty of refpiration, pain in
the fide, or fome other fymptom takes
place, and denotes the peculiar influence
of the difeafe on fome or more of the
vifcera: and, that to thefe fymptoms fucceed thofe which are the figns of a languid

guid and nearly extinguished circulation.
It is therefore essential to sound and suc-
cessful practice, that the physician be mi-
nutely informed of all the signs that lead
to point out the healthy state of the viscera, and of the principal organs of the
circulation; and likewise those which
on the other hand, indicate the more or
less baneful influence of Acute Diseases;
on those organs, or on the viscera. These
latter ones constantly announce more or
less of danger, whereas the others enliven
our hopes. These signs, when drawn
from exact observation of the different
symptoms of Acute Diseases that terminate in death, or that end in a cure, become the most solid basis of the Prognostic in these cases; and it is therefore
to those signs that we shall devote the
First Section of our work.

When a patient is attacked with an
acute fever, and cured by the resources of
nature alone, and without the assistance
of art; we almost always observe, that
this happy termination of the disease is

due

due to fome evacuation, or to fome critical external abfcefs , or to fome eruption,
by means of which nature feems to carry
out of the circulation, the morbific matter
which had occafioned the difeafe. Attentive phyficians likewife obferve the
fame thing to happen to almoft all the patients in this way who come under their
care.

THESE evacuations, or abfceffes, or e-
ruptions, which take place in the courfe
of acute difeafes, are not always, however,
equally falutary. In fome circumftances
they announce danger ,in others they even
denote the death of the patient to be at
hand. It is therefore of importance to
know and to be able to diftinguifh the force
and value of all the various figns that have
any affinity with thefe evacuations, abfceffes, or eruptions: which, according to
the difference of their qualities or of the
fymptoms that accompany them, announce
either a cure, or more or lefs of danger.
Thefe figns which will be the fubject of
our fecond fection, not only ferve to eft a
blifh the prognoftic ; but are likewife ufeful

ful in directing us to the proper treatment
of the fick. The phyfician, who is igno-
rant of, or inattentive to them, will often
be liable to the moft dangerous errors,
by depending, at improper feafons, and
without reafon, on the refources of nature,
or by difturbing her by ufelefs, and perhaps noxious remedies, at the time when
fhe is favourably exerting herfelf to terminate the difeafe.

In the third feétion we mean to colleét
together many figns which are very ufeful to be known; but which cannot be
eafily arranged in either the firft or the
fecond feétion.

THE fourth feétion will contain the
prognoftic figns that are peculiar to inflammation and abfcefs of the breaft, and to
fome other acute difeafes.

SECTION

SECTION I.

CHAP. I.

Of the signs which indicate the state of the cir-
culating powers; and of the prognostics
to be derived from them.

§ I. IT is of advantage, in acute fevers, to
find the pulse yielding, equal, and free;
and that with respect to strength, it be not
very different from the natural pulse.

§ II. The pulse which is at the same
time frequent, small, soft, weak and often
unequal, and which persists in this character,
is habitual to pestilential and malignant fevers, and likewise to the inflammation of the breast, angina and dysentery
which we name malignant. (* 1.) It announces danger.

§ III. When

§ III. WHEN the pulse from being free
and open (*développé*), with some degree
of strength and even hardness, becomes
small, soft, and weak, the sign is an unfavourable one.   We may fear that this disease will soon terminate in death.   (* 2.)
On the other hand we may speak more favourably of what is to happen when the
pulse from being in this latter state becomes
more strong and open.

§ IV. A VERY small, weak pulse announces imminent danger.   The creeping
and thread like pulse, is the forerunner of
death.

§ V. THE empty pulse (*pouls vuide*);
for so we call that pulse which with
the sensation of extent, seems at the same
time to be soft and weak, forebodes imminent danger.   (* 3.)

§ VI. ALTHOUGH the state of the pulse
may be alarming, we are not however to
suppose that death is at hand, unless the
attitude (§ x v and seq.), and physiognomy
§ XXIV

(§ xxiv and feq.) of the patient corroborate the prognoftic.

§ VII. The intermitting pulfe if it has ftrength, is not fo dangerous in acute difeafes, as the ancients fuppofed it to be: It is no alarming fymptom in old perfons: It is fometimes a forerunner of falutary diarrhœa: It does not even forbid venæfection, if the other circumftances feem to indicate the evacuation.

§ VIII. Amongst the variety of acute difeafes, it fometimes happens, that the pulfe does not beat with more frequency, or is even flower, than in health. This character of the pulfe cannot therefore, on fuch occafions, fenfibly influence the prognoftic; which we muft derive from the ftrength or weaknefs of the pulfe, and from all the other fymptoms of the difeafe.

§ IX. Bilious, acrid matter, or worms, irritating the inteftinal canal; paffions of the mind; hemorrhage; vomiting; or a
fudden

ſudden and copious diarrhoea, may occaſion a temporary weakneſs and irregularity of the pulſe, which ought not to alarm
us.

§ X. In a great number of caſes, the
prognoſtic, if founded ſolely on the pulſe,
would deceive us. We are therefore
not to confine ourſelves to the conſidera-
tion of the pulſe alone : we muſt carefully
and attentively examine and deliberate on
all the ſigns that the diſeaſe preſents to us;
and after having reflected on theſe and
all that preceded the attack, we muſt form
our prognoſtic by combining all thoſe con-
ſiderations together.

§ XI. If, after ſitting up for ſome time,
a patient feels himſelf faint, the phyſician
is not to be alarmed.

§ XII. The faintneſs, which at the beginning of an acute fever, is occaſioned
by bilious matter, or worms irritating the
ſtomach, is in no way dangerous.

§ XIII.

§ XIII EVEN fyncope, tho' always more or lefs alarming, has not ufually any bad confequences, when occafioned by the above caufes (§ XI, XII.), or by the paffions of the mind.

§ XIV. BUT the faintnefs, and above all, the fyncope, which fometimes appears in the courfe of an acute fever, without feeming in any way to depend on either of the above caufes (§ XI, XII, XIII), are to be confidered as very dangerous fymptoms. It is then to be feared left a frefh fyncope fhould fuddenly put an end to the patient. (*4.)

§ XV. To judge properly of the ftate of a patient's ftrength, we fhould attentively confider what are the attitudes he takes and is able to fupport.

§ XVI. IT is in general a very favourable fign, when the patient is able to get up to fatisfy his wants; and when he is able to fit up for fome time without much inconvenience; or that if he keeps his bed
altogether

altogether. That he lie in it on one fide, with his legs, thighs and body fomewhat bent, becaufe this is an attitude which fuppofes fome degree of ftrength, and is familiar to perfons in health. *Hip.* 9.

§ XVII. If he lies conftantly on his back, this attitude is the effect and the fign of great weaknefs. It ufually occurs in the moft alarming acute fevers, and concurs with the other fymptoms in pointing out their danger. *Hip.* 10.

§ XVIII. If in this attitude the patient keeps his legs and arms fpread; his hands, feet, neck, and breaft bare, altho' thefe parts feel fenfibly cold to the touch; thefe fymptoms, of diftrefs (§ xx), and infenfibility, add to the unfavourablenefs of the Prognoftic (§ xvii). *Hip.* 12.

§ XIX. If the patient is continually fliding down towards the foot of the bed, fo that the affiftants are frequently obliged to raife him to his pillow, we may argue an exceffive weaknefs, which is to be

D con-

confidered as a moſt alarming ſymptom. *Hip*. 11.

§ XX. THE anxiety, or in other
words, the internal uneaſineſs which
obliges the patient to be inceſſantly varying his poſition, is very commonly the
forerunner of death.   When this happens,
the anxiety has uſually been preceded,
and continues to be accompanied, by the
moſt alarming ſymptoms; ſuch as a very
bad pulſe, the *facies hippocratica* (§ xxv,
xxvii), coldneſs of the extremities, cold
ſweats, exceſſive weakneſs and inſenſi-
bility. *Hip*. 13, 14.

§ XXI. IF, the patient, tormented by
a conſtant internal ſenſation of heat, is
inceſſantly throwing the bed cloaths from
off his breaſt, we may conclude this to
be a moſt fatal ſymptom, which precedes
and even accompanies the agonies of
death.

§ XXII. BUT when this anxiety takes
place at the beginning of an Acute
Diſeaſe,

Difeafe, without having been preceded or
even accompanied with any other alarming fymptom, the Prognoftic will be more
favourable.   In this cafe it will often
depend on a fimple affection of the ftomach from irritating bile, worms, &c.
which ceafes the moment it is freed
from thefe caufes, either by means of art
or nature.

§ XXIII. If from the firft onfet of an
acute fever, the ftrength of the patient
appears to be much weakened, altho' the
fever is not violent, nor has been preceded by great pain or evacuations, yet
we may conclude, that the fever will be
of the malignant kind. *Hip*. 15.

§ XXIV. It is of advantage for the
patient's phyfiognomy to be nearly in a
natural ftate; that his look be firm and
clear; that his face be not meagre, and
deprived of its flefh; that his complexion
be not very different from what it was
in health; that his lips preferve their
natural colour, and that they be clofed

even

even while the patient fleeps, unlefs his noftrils are ftopped, or that he is accuftomed to fleep with his mouth open. *Hip.* 16.

§ XXV. But if his nofe appears lengthened, his eyes funk, his temples hollow, and the fkin of his forehead dry and diftended: if at the fame time his ears are cold, dry, and drawn back; his complexion exceedingly pale or faturnine; his look, languifhing; and his lower lip hanging down. Such a change as this in the features, is a proof of exceffive weaknefs, and announces the moft imminent danger. *Hip.* 16.

XXVI. These fymptoms, however, are lefs formidable, when they appear at the beginning of an acute fever: efpecially when they have been preceded and occafioned by any excefs; by a violent diarrhœa; by a laborious and obftinate vomiting; or by a confiderable hemorrhage: in either of thefe cafes, the change in the phyfiognomy ufually

disappears

difappears within four and twenty hours,
and fometimes in lefs time. But if, independent of any of thefe caufes, we
obferve fuch figns (§ xxv.) towards the
clofe of an Acute Difeafe, which has
before been attended with the moft alarming fymptoms, and exhaufted the ftrength
of the patient, we may conclude that he
is near his end. *Hip.* 17.

§ XXVII. In this laft cafe his phyfiognomy often affords other figns which
confirm the fatality of the Prognoftic. His
look is fometimes wholly extinguifhed,
or he directs it in an oppofite direction to
the voice that calls him; his eyes feem
filled with tears or they appear to be
foul, fixed and jutting out, or inceffantly
agitated with fudden and convulfive motions; or elfe remaining open, the pupil
is wholly, or in fome degree hid under
the upper eye lid. Sometimes even the
cornea becomes faded and tarnifhed; the
pupil dilates itfelf; the mouth is turned
awry, or open, and the lips are pale and
cold:

cold: fometimes, to all thefe, are added marks of lividity about the temples, and around the lips. *Hip.* 18 & feq.

§ XXVIII. The livid complexion of the ends of the fingers and nails, a permanent coldnefs of the extremities, cold fweats, and rattling in the throat, are fymptoms that are frequently attendant on the unhappy figns we have defcribed. This melancholy fcene is at length clofed by a refpiration, which every moment becomes lefs frequent, till the patient breathes his laft figh, with horrid convulfions in the mufcles of the mouth.

§ XXIX. A long habit, of attending carefully at the bed-fide of the fick, to all the figns, that the phyfiognomy, the attitude, and the refpiration of the patient are able to afford, furnifhes the experienced Phyfician with that mafterly eye, which enables him to appreciate, with great readinefs, the figns of

this

this kind, and to draw from them **a**
Prognoſtic, which ſometimes appears to
us to be not leſs wonderful by the
propriety of judgement, than by the
facility, with which it ſeems to be
made.

CHAP.

C H A P. II.

Of the signs which indicate the sound state of the viscera, or which prove them to be more or less affected.

§ XXX. IT is of advantage, in Acute Diseases, for the belly to be soft, as in the natural state; and at the same time, neither tumid nor painful. *Hip.* 23.

§ XXXI. If the volume of the abdomen seems increased; if, when gently tapped, it resounds like a drum: we learn from these signs, the flatulent distension of the abdomen.

§ XXXII.

§ XXXII. The Prognostic to be derived from it, will be very different, according to its different degrees.

§ XXXIII. If this distension takes place only in some particular part of the lower belly; or if, altho' seemingly extending through the whole of it, it is only inconsiderable; and if, at the same time, it is not accompanied by pains which might lead to suspect the inflammation of some of the abdominal viscera, there is nothing formidable in the appearance. We every day see it happen in Acute Diseases which terminate happily, and without any appearance of danger.

§ XXXIV. But if the abdomen becomes enormously tumid, and distended with *flatus*, the appearance is then of alarming portent. *Hip.* 25. It is usually accompanied by a number of other symptoms, which equally announce, either very imminent danger, or the approach of death. (* 5.)

E, § XXXV,

§ XXXV. The eruption of flatus at the mouth, caufes this diftenfion to ceafe in the epigaftric region.

§ XXXVI. That which is feated in either of the Hypochondria, is commonly diffipated by copious ftools and borborygmata; whether thefe evacuations are fpontaneous or occafioned by the ufe of purgatives.

§ XXXVII. The pains, which in Acute Difeafes, chance to attack any particular part of the lower belly, afford a very different Prognoftic, according as they are more or lefs increafed or unaffected by preffure.

§ XXXVIII. The pains, which are not increafed by preffure, are occafioned by acrid, bilious matter; by flatus; or by worms, that irritate the ftomach and inteftines. Pains of this fort are not alarming.

§ XXXIX.

§ XXXIX. The same causes, however, (§ xxxviii.) altho' seated in the lower belly, sometimes occasion pains, which are by the patient referred to the breast. And they likewise, sometimes, excite cough and difficulty of breathing. (* 6.)

§ XL. If, during the course of an acute fever, a patient complains of pains and of an irregular pricking sensation within the abdomen or thorax; *Hip.* 45. we may presume that he has, and will evacuate, round worms. The known character of an epidemic disease, often confirms such a suspicion, and reduces it almost to certainty.

§ XLI. If, the patient complains that he feels something rising from time to time into his thorax, so as to threaten suffocation, we may be almost assured that this symptom is occasioned by worms irritating the upper orifice of the stomach, and rising even into the oeso-phagus.

§ XLII.

§ XLII. A PAIN, more or lefs acute, at the ftomach, and particularly at the hollow of the ftomach, is another fymptom which we pretty frequently obferve in acute fevers.

§ XLIII. IF neither palpitation, nor a flight compreffion of the ftomach fenfibly increafe this pain ; we may fuppofe that it depends on bilious, acrid matter, or on worms; and therefore are not to be alarmed by it.

§ XLIV. BUT if the flighteft preffure adds to the pain and renders it infupportable; we may conclude it to be inflammatory. In this cafe it will afford a very unfavourable Prognoftic. *Hip.* 44. It will then likewife be accompanied with other fymptoms, which will corroborate the idea of great danger.

§ XLV. IF, during the courfe of an Acute Difeafe, there comes on a pain in one or other of the hypochondria, or in fome other part of the lower belly, and
which

which is not fensibly increafed by compreffion; we may fuppofe it to be feated
in fome inteftine diftended by flatus,
or irritated by bilious matter, **or by
worms.**

§ XLVI. If, after an exact palpitation,
we are able to trace the figure of a diftended inteftine, and any noife is felt or
heard in the bowels, at the fame time;
we can no longer doubt that the pain is
produced by flatus.

§ XLVII. Pains of this fort are neither
dangerous nor durable. Evacuations
by ftool, difcharge of air by the anus,
and fometimes fimple borborygmata, are
found to diffipate them. *Hip*. 41.

§ XLVIII. But if in the courfe of an
acute fever, there appears a gliftening,
painful tumefaction of fome part of the
lower belly; and the pain that accompanies it, becomes fenfibly more acute, on
the flighteft preffure: and if it is rendered
infupportable by making a little more
com-

compreffion; we may be convinced that
this part is in a ftate of inflammation, and
indeed we fhall ufually find it accompanied by other formidable fymptoms,
Hip. 28, 29, 30, 31, 32.

§ XLIX. This fymptom may be difcovered even in comatofe affections, by
the diftortion that appears in the countenance of the patient, whenever we
carry our hand to the inflamed part.

§ L. This fymptom, tho' commonly a
mortal one, is, however, not always fo.
Sometimes, tho' rarely, tumours of this
fort degenerate into abfcefs, more efpecially when they are feated in the liver,
Hip. 31, 32.

§ LI. We have reafon to fufpect that
the difeafe will take this turn, when the
fymptom continues to perfift, without
the concurrence of the other fymptoms
that conftantly announce the approach
of Death. *Hip.* 31, 32.

§ LII.

§ LII. When an abſceſs of this ſort is actually formed, it is to be wiſhed, that it may ſoon appear externally, and maniſeſt itſelf by that kind of oedematous ſtate of the common integuments, which, in deep abſceſſes, announces them to be making their way outwards; and that the fluctuation may ſoon be ſufficiently ſenſible for us to evacuate the matter. *Hip.* 38, 39.

§ LIII. On carrying the hand careſully over the abdomen, in patients attacked with acute fevers, we ſometimes, tho' rarely, perceive a large, gliſtening and firm tumour, but without any marks of inflammation or pain, in the umbilical region. Tumours of this ſort do not ſeem to be dangerous. They are commonly diſſipated by copious evacuations by ſtool; whether they be ſpontaneous, or determined by means of purgative medicines.

§ LIV. The Aſcites, which ſometimes takes place in the courſe of an acute fever,

fever, is ufually the effect of an inflammation of the bowels, that is generally mortal. (* 7.) *Hip*. 43.

§ LV. WHEN the patient breathes, as he did in health; and is able to make a deep infpiration without feeling any inconvenience, or pain, or excitement to cough: we may not only conclude, that neither the lungs, nor pleura, are injured; but likewife, that the abdominal vifcera are in a good ftate, and that no dangerous change has as yet taken place in the functions of the circulatory organs. No fign, therefore, can be more comforting and confolatory than this is, whenever we obferve it in acute fevers. *Hip*. 46.

§ LVI. ALTHO' the refpiration fhould appear to be pretty free; yet, if the patient is unable to make a deep infpiration, without feeling an uneafinefs, or irritation, or pain in fome part of the breaft, it proves, that the thorax is not abfolutely untouched, and ought, therefore, to lead the phyfician to inquire,

with

with the utmost care, whether the lungs suffer only from a simple irritation, or whether there is not reason to suspect some more serious affection.

§ LVII. An acute fever, renders the respiration more frequent and laborious, than in a natural state. The Prognostic of this kind of respiration, does not differ from that of the fever, which occasions it.

§ LVIII. If, during the course of an acute idiopathic fever, we observe symptoms of pleurisy, or peripneumony; such a complication can afford only an unfavourable Prognostic. *Hip*. 47.

§ LIX. The inflammations of the breast, however, which occasionally take place in the course of acute fevers, are not, in general, so fatal, as those, which, in fevers of the same kind, affect the abdominal viscera. (8.)

F   LX.

§ LX. The exacerbations, of continued remittent fevers, are often announced, and even preceded, by a vexatious cough.

§ LXI. The cough, and even the difficulty of breathing, when they take place only at the beginning of the exacerbation, often originate more from the irritation of bile in the ſtomach, than from any morbid affection of the breaſt.

§ LXII. When a patient lies with greater inconvenience on one ſide, than on the other; we are to conſider, that this ſymptom may belong to different diſeaſes; as, for example, to an inflamed ſtate of one of the lobes of the lungs; or to an effuſion of pus, or of ſerum, into one of the cavities of the thorax; we ſhall deſcribe the Diagnoſtic, and Prognoſtic of each of theſe different caſes, in the fourth ſection, when we come to ſpeak of inflammations of the breaſt, and their effects.

§ LXIII.

§ LXIII. If the patient speaks hastily, and unintelligibly, it proves that he is either delirious, or has his respiration much incommoded. In this last case, the patient is unable to converse long at a time; his words are uttered much quicker at the close, than at the beginning, of a phrase. If this symptom happens to be the effect of delirium, it may be known by the signs (§ 76. 78, 79.) which characterize it.

§ LXIV. A slow and laborious respiration, usually accompanies comatose affection and silent delirium. *Hip.* 48.

§ LXV. Plaintful respiration, during sleep, is always to be considered as an alarming symptom, unless it is the transitory effect of an uneasy dream. While the patient is awake, the Prognostic from this symptom, can be formed only by comparing it with the temperament, and disposition of the patient. If he is delicate, tender of himself, impatient of pain, and accustomed to exaggerate the

F 2   least

leaſt ſuffering, we ſhall be leſs alarmed, than if he is naturally robuſt, and of a patient temper.

§ LXVI. A small, and frequent reſpiration, is an alarming ſymptom; whether it depends wholly on the exceſſive weakneſs of the patient, or whether it be the effect of an acute pain in the breaſt, or of a conſiderable tumefaction of the lungs, or of an acute pain in any part of the lower belly. *Hip.* 47.

§ LXVII. The reſpiration, which is at once ſmall, quick, and laborious, is ſtill more dangerous.

§ LXVIII. When the reſpiration in Acute Diſeaſes, is ſo laborious, as to be performed with ſhort breathing, and with the manifeſt action of the muſcles of the neck and breaſt, and even of the alæ of the noſe; we may conclude that death is at hand.

§ LXIX.

§ LXIX. The respiration cut off, *spiratio luctuosa, spiritus offendens*, is a most alarming symptom. *Hip.* 51, 52.

§ LXX. If, in the course of an acute fever, the patient is suddenly attacked with an extreme difficulty of breathing; or is oppressed, so as to require to be supported by pillows, and to sit up, the Prognostic will be very unfavourable. This symptom, particularly takes place in inflammatory diseases of the breast. (§ ccccxli.) *Hip.* 53.

§ LXXI. A RATTLING in the throat, indicates the agony of death. It is accompanied by all the other signs of death.

§ LXXII. It is perhaps superfluous to observe, that the physician is not to confound with this last symptom, the noise in the throat, which sometimes happens in inflammations of the breast, when the patient expectorates with difficulty. He

must

muſt, indeed, be a novice in phyſic, who
makes ſuch a miſtake.

§ LXXIII. Slow reſpiration, the in-
tervals of which, are every moment
more and more lengthened out, is the
immediate forerunner of death.

§ LXXIV. It ſometimes happens, and
eſpecially in comatoſe affections, that this
kind of reſpiration alone, and without
any rattling in the throat, announces the
death of the patient.

§ LXXV. It is of advantage in Acute
Diſeaſes, for the patient to enjoy fully,
the faculties of his ſoul; that there be
nothing changed in his ſentiments, or
actions; that his countenance be clear,
and free from any ſickly heavineſs; that
he be not without ſleep, but that the
ſleep he enjoys, be tranquil and refreſhing. All theſe ſigns are favourable ones.
We may conclude from them, that neither
the brain, nor the nervous ſyſtem, are
affected by the diſeaſe. *Hip.* 57.

§ LXXVI.

§ LXXVI. Neither errors of judgement in familiar matters, nor manifest errors of the senses, nor an irregular imagination are the sole marks of delirium; every change in the voice, discourse, gestures, actions, and even in the countenance of the patient, proves that his soul is no longer in her natural seat, and are sufficiently characteristic of delirium, to the eye of the attentive and experienced physician. *Hip*. 60, 61, 64, 65, 66.

§ LXXVII. We are not to confound with true delirium, the reveries of the patient, who either when sleeping, or half asleep, mutters through his teeth, or holds some unreasonable discourse. Nothing is more common, than a symptom of this sort, even in the mildest fevers; and nothing is less alarming, provided the patient, on being roused and interrogated, looks and answers in a natural manner.

§ LXXVIII.

§ LXXVIII. Violent and obstinate head ach, redness of the face and eyes, humming and tingling in the ears, (*tinnitus aurium*) together with watchfulness, and limpid urine, are the symptoms which commonly precede and announce delirium. *Hip.* 58, 62, 63.

§ LXXIX. If the patient's imagination is more lively than usual; if he is loquacious, speaks hastily, and has a bold, piercing look, with a certain brilliancy about his eyes; we may conclude, that the delirium has taken place. *Hip.* 58.

§ LXXX. The gay and gentle delirium, which is neither furious nor silent, and which is accompanied neither with comatose affection, nor with any other bad symptom, is often more alarming than dangerous. (* 9.) *Hip.* 67.

§ LXXXI. There are some persons, who from a particular constitution, are easily affected with delirium, whenever they are attacked with a small fever.

In

In fuch fubjects, delirium is, in general, a much lefs dangerous and alarming fymptom, than it is in perfons who are not difpofed to it by temperament. *Hip.* 68.

§ LXXXII. DELIRIUM is, in general, more frequent, and lefs dangerous, in the difeafes of young perfons, (*adole-fcentes*) than in adults, old people, and infants. (* 10.) *Hip.* 68.

§ LXXXIII. WE obferve the furious delirium, only in the difeafes of young people.

§ LXXXIV. IT is of advantage for the delirium, to correfpond nearly with the degree of fever : and that it increafe or diminifh with it.

§ LXXXV. BUT if when the pulfe, and the vis vitæ diminifh, the delirium does not likewife abate, but even increafes, the Prognoftic will be a very unfavour-able one.

G § LXXXVI.

§ LXXXVI. It is a good sign, when the patient, after being tormented with delirium, at length falls asleep; and that this sleep, by being gentle and refreshing, and of sufficient length, removes the delirium.----Such a change, usually announces the cure. *Hip.* 69.

§ LXXXVII. Every phrenitic delirium, announces great danger; whether it be dull and silent, or raging and talkative. *Hip.* 73.

§ LXXXVIII. If when the patient is silently delirious, his trembling hands are incessantly employed in picking the bed clothes, or the neighbouring wall, he is in the greatest danger. *Hip.* 71, 72.

§ LXXXIX. It is disagreeable, and indeed unhappy, when the patient's delirium being confined to objects that are essential to himself, prevents him from drinking, and taking nourishment, and in short, from doing whatever is necessary to his cure. *Hip.* 74.

§ XC.

§ XC. Delirium, when accompanied with *fubfultus tendinum*, is always dangerous. We have ftill more to fear when delirious patients are inceffantly agitated by an exceffive fenfibility, or by fear. (* 11.) *Hip.* 70. 75.

§ XCI. When delirium is combined with convulfive motions, either in the wrifts, or eyes, or mufcles of the face, neck, or head; it is mortal.

§ XCII. Nor are epileptic convulfions, and the grinding of the teeth, which take place in phrenitic delirium, lefs certainly followed by death. Extreme weaknefs; tremor; bad pulfe; convulfive motions, foulnefs, and rednefs of the eyes; vomiting of dark, black matter; the tongue dry, parched and trembling; the lips feparated; the fore teeth covered with a vifcid, dry and dark coloured matter; together with an extreme change in the features of the face; thefe are the fymptoms which ufually accompany delirium, when

G 2

it

it has a tendency to death. *Hip.* 77. & feq.

§ XCIII. If this phrenitic delirium ceafes without this reafon, that is, if the patient refumes his fenfes without this change having been occafioned by any critical evacuation, or depofition, the dangerous fymptoms which accompanied it, ftill continuing; the death of the patient is at hand. (§ cclxxxvii.)

§ XCIV. If, when the patient has fhewn his tongue to a phyfician, he forgets to withdraw it again ; or if when he has called for the chamber pot, he omits to make water, &c. thefe marks of abfence, or diftraction, prove that he is either delirious, or comatofe. *Hip.* 82.

§ XCV. It is of advantage, if he preferves his phyfical and moral fenfibility ; and is affected, as in his natural ftate, both by heat and cold, as well as by all the other caufes that may be liable to make

impreffions

imprefſions on his ſenſes ; it will be well too, if his mind continues to preſerve its faculties, in circumſtances which may be expected to intereſt, or excite emotions in it.

§ XCVI. But if the patient has the mouth and tongue parched, together with great heat and dryneſs of the body, and yet complains not of thirſt; if we find his hands, or his feet, or both, out of bed, altho' they feel cold ; if he goes to ſtool, and likewiſe voids his urine, inſenſibly ; if he ſeems to have no concern in whatever is going on around him, and if he looks with indifference, during the moſt diſtreſsful ſcenes; we may conclude, that his brain is grievouſly affected, and that he is wholly deprived of ſenſibility. Such a ſtate, cannot take place, without announcing the greateſt danger. *Hip.* 83, & ſeq.

§ XCVII. It is a good ſign, (tho' it ſeldom happens) in Acute Diſeaſes, when the patient ſleeps in the night, and lies awake

awake during the day, as he uſed to do when in health.

§ XCVIII. It is ſalutary, however, when he ſleeps during a few hours in a tranquil manner, ſo that when he wakes he finds himſelf refreſhed. The more he approaches to his natural ſtate, in this reſpect, the more favourable will be our Prognoſtic. *Hip.* 88, & ſeq.

§ XCIX. Watchfulness, uſually pre-cedes, announces, and accompanies deli-rium. (§ lxxviii.)

§ C. Uneasy, plaintive ſleep, diſturbed by diſagreeable and fatiguing dreams, and which exhauſts, inſtead of refreſhing the patient, altho' it is not to be arranged with the more grievous ſymptoms of the diſeaſe, yet it ought to excite the atten-tion of the phyſician, when he is conſi-dering the character, and progreſs of the fever, and endeavouring to form a Prog-noſtic, from all the ſymptoms it affords.

§ CI,

§ CI. Iꜰ the patient's sleep is disturbed by unusual grinding of the teeth, and wakes frequently, on a sudden, and as it were frightened, we have reason to fear some epileptic convulsive attack ; especially if this happens to a child ; and the more so, if the patient's cheeks are flushed, and his eyes fixed and brilliant. *Hip*. 103.

§ CII. Iꜰ the patient, who sleeps more than in a natural state, and even soundly, does, however, when roused and thoroughly awakened, appear to have a clear countenance, and to answer readily and with propriety, to the questions we put to him ; such a sleep as this, is often merely the effect of a somewhat smart fever. It does in no way prove the brain to be grievously affected ; and therefore ought not to be confounded. with comatose affection.

§ CIII. Bᴜᴛ if we are unable to rouse the patient ; or if, when roused, he wakes with difficulty, has a stupid, unmeaning
countenance,

countenance, and feems hardly, or not at all, to conceive the queftions we put to him, and more efpecially if he returns no anfwer, or if his anfwers indicate delirium; and while we are fpeaking to him, fleep feems inceffantly to be over-powering him; if he feems to be forget-ful, or infenfible; (§ xcvi.) we may con-clude from thefe figns, that he has a true comatofe affection, and this cannot be without danger. *Hip*. 91.

§ CIV. Comatose affections, in acute fevers, are in general, fomewhat lefs dan-gerous, and more frequent in adults, and perfons of more advanced age, than in younger fubjects.

§ CV. Their danger is nearly in pro-portion to their degree. *Carus* is ufually fatal. *Hip*. 92, 93, 94, 95.

§ CVI. Comatose, intermittent, and remittent fevers, the paroxyfms of which begin with horripilatio, yield more eafily to the bark, and are, in general, lefs

dangerous

dangerous than comatofe remittents, which affume the type of continued fevers.

§ CVII. If, in fevers of this laft kind, the pulfe from being frequent and open (*developpé*) during the remiffion, becomes very quick, foft; weak, and unequal in the paroxyfms: if, at each paroxyfm, this fymptom feems to increafe, as well as the ftrength and continuance of the heavinefs the patients complain of in thefe cafes; we have every reafon to believe that the difeafe will be mortal.

§ CVIII. This unfavourable Prognoftic, will be the more confirmed, if we have unfuccefsfully employed the bark, to fupprefs or diminifh the violence of the paroxyfms.

§ CIX. An inability to fwallow; bad pulfe; laboured, ftertorous, or very rare, refpiration; convulfive motions in the fingers, or wrifts, or in the mufcles of the head or face; *Hip.* 97. a vomiting of

H   atrabilis,

atrabilis, and permanent coldnefs of the extremities; *Hip*. 96. The under jaw hanging down; livid complexion of the nails and ends of the fingers; marks of lividity around the lips and temples, are the unhappy fymptoms which, in cafes of comatofe affection, announce, that it is about to terminate in death.

§ CX. The lethargy is fometimes fympathetic, and dependent on pulmonary inflammation or abfcefs. If the patient efcapes in this cafe, the diforder is ufually followed by an expectoration of pus. *Hip*. 100.

§ CXI. *Subfultus tendinum*, is a frequent fymptom in malignant fevers, and in other Acute Difeafes, which partake of the fame character. We likewife obferve this affection after confiderable wounds, and compound fractures, when the cafes take a bad turn and excite a fever of the fame kind. This fubfultus may, therefore, always be confidered as announcing danger. (¯ 12.)

§ CXII.

§ CXII. The Prognoſtic, in this caſe, will be more or leſs favorable, in proportion as the ſubſultus is more or leſs violent; it will be neceſſary, however, to conſider all the other ſymptoms, and likewiſe the age of the patient, before we form our opinion.

§ CXIII. This ſymptom is more familiar to, and likewiſe leſs dangerous in youth, than it is in infants, adults, and old perſons.

§ CXIV. If, during the courſe of an acute fever, that is accompanied with the moſt dangerous ſymptoms, we obſerve, that the thumb of either hand, is from time to time, affeĉted with ſudden and convulſive motions; or, if we obſerve ſimilar ſpaſms in the wriſts, or in ſome part of the face, or, as it ſometimes happens, in the muſcles, which move the head upon the neck: ſuch a ſymptom announces a ſpeedy and certain death.

H 2

§ CXV.

§ CXV. WE fometimes fee, (efpecially in the comatofe affections of infants) fimilar convulfive motions in the globe of the eye.

§ CXVI. THIS laſt fymptom is equally fatal, when it comes on at the clofe of any difeafe, whether acute or chronic. Altho' it is always very alarming, yet there is not fo much to be feared from it, when it appears at the beginning of an acute fever, or of the fmall pox, during the lethargic ſtate that ufually follows the convulfive affection, which is commonly a forerunner of the eruption in this latter difeafe; we know it to be a frequent fymptom in young fubjects.

§ CXVII. THE epileptic convulſions which come on at the clofe of an Acute Difeafe, are fatal, and as well to children as to adults. *Hip.* 107, 108, 109, 110. Thefe convulfions are fometimes preceded by a fenfation of tenfion in the mufcles of the neck, and by a pain, unaccompanied by tumour or rednefs, in the throat. *Hip.*

Hip. 112, 113, 114. (* 13.) Thofe which come on at the end of a chronic difeafe, are equally baneful to patients of every age. (* 14.)

§ CXVIII. Although convulfions of this fort, are always alarming, they are, however, much lefs dangerous, when they appear at the beginning of an acute fever.

§ CXIX. Setting apart the cafes juft now mentioned (§ cxvii), we may obferve, that thefe convulfions are more frequent in children under feven years of age, than in older fubjects. *Hip.* 103.

§ CXX. An epileptic patient may, in the courfe of an acute fever, have one or more attacks of epilepfy, which as they are the effects of a chronic and habitual complaint, cannot fenfibly interfere with the Prognoftic in an Acute Difeafe.

§ CXXI. Women, and efpecially fuch as are delicate, vapourifh, and hyfterical, are,

are, in general, more eafily fufceptible
of convulfive affection, than other fubjects, and ufually with lefs danger.

§ CXXII. Convulsions, occafioned by
enormous hemorrhage, or purging, or by
pain, announce the moft imminent danger. *Hip.* 116, 117, 118, 119, 120.

§ CXXIII. When a patient is perfe-
cuted with exceffive and long continued
pain, it is to be feared, left he be attacked
with epileptic convulfions, and even apoplexy. *Hip.* 98. (* 15.)

§ CXXIV. If, hiccup comes on during
the courfe of an acute fever, we ought
particularly to confider what were the
fymptoms which preceded and accompanied it, and by what caufes it feems to be
excited.

§ CXXV. When hiccup is accompanied by no other alarming fymptom, it
is often merely the effect of bilious, acid,
or other humours, or worms, irritating
the

the ſtomach; and in ſuch caſes, a vomiting, or copious ſtools, will remove the
complaint. Sometimes a draught of
diluting liquor is ſufficient to carry it
off.

§ CXXVI. Iꜰ the other ſymptoms denote the hiccup to depend on the inflammation of any abdominal viſcus, it is
fatal. It likewiſe affords a very unfavourable Prognoſtic in Iliac paſſion,
ſtrangulated Hernia, and Dyſentery.

§ CXXVII. Tʜᴇ hiccup which comes
on at the cloſe of an acute fever, preceded and accompanied by other moſt
dangerous ſymptoms, the patient being
at the ſame time in a debilitated ſtate, is
mortal.

§ CXXVIII. Tʜᴇ ſame may be ſaid
of that which follows profuſe hemorrhage.
Hip. 118.

§ CXXIX. Hɪᴄᴄᴜᴘ coming on in an
acute fever, after a ſymptomatic vomiting

ing of greenish or atrabilious matter, announces death to be at hand. *Hip.* 101.

§ CXXX. TETANOS is very reasonably confidered as one of thofe difeafes, which are the moft acute in their progrefs, and the moft generally fatal in their event. *Hip.* 123.

§ CXXXI. WHEN a wounded patient feels a painful tenfion in the mufcles of his neck, or is unable to open his mouth, thefe fymptoms announce tetanos, and of courfe, the great danger there is of fpeedy death. *Hip.* 114.

§ CXXXII. I HAVE before fpoken (§ XCII. CI.) of the Prognoftic to be derived from the grinding of the teeth.

§ CXXXIII. DEAFNESS is a fymptom that is particularly obferved in malignant fevers.

§ CXXXIV.

§ CXXXIV. COMING on at the beginning of an acute fever, it may help to
characterize it. It will be found, however, to be in general, the forerunner of
phrenitic delirium, and of the moſt grievous ſymptoms.

§ CXXXV. THE deafneſs, which
comes on at the cloſe of an Acute Diſeaſe, is fatal, if it is ſymptomatic. But
more commonly, at this period of the
diſeaſe, it is critical. In this latter caſe,
as it increaſes, the patient appears to be
more and more relieved.

§ CXXXVI. THIS deafneſs uſually goes
off by degrees, in the convaleſcent ſtate.
Sometimes, however, it reſiſts every remedy, and the patient remains deaf.

§ CXXXVII. MALIGNANT fevers likewiſe terminate, ſometimes by Gutta ſe-
rena, or by loſs of memory, or by imbe-
cility. Theſe affections, like the former
one, commonly (tho' not always) diſap-
pear as the patient recovers.

I   § CXXXVIII.

§ CXXXVIII. BLINDNESS, coming on at the clofe of an acute fever, (the other fatal figns continuing,) is ufually a fign of death.

§ CXXXIX. IN infants, this fymptom (§ cxxxviii.) is eafily known, even in cafes of lethargic, apopleƈtic affeƈtion, by an exceffive dilatation of the pupil.

§ CXL. IF, on approaching a candle to the eye of a child, fo affeƈted, we obferve no contraƈtion of the pupil, we may conclude that the eye has totally loft its fenfibility.

§ CXLI. THIS fymptom is often com-plicated with a convulfive motion of the globe of the eye.

§ CXLII. SUCH figns (§ cxl, cxli.) as thefe, announce a fpeedy death. There is one cafe, however, in which they are not fo conftantly fatal; and that is, when they take place in the comatofe ftate, which fometimes follows the epileptic convul-fions

fions at the beginning of an acute fever, and particulary, of the fmall pox.

§ CXLIII. Palsy of the tongue, hemiplegia, or crofs palfy, (*Paralyfie croifee*) (* 16.) coming on during the courfe of a malignant fever, and being purely fymptomatical, announce the greateft danger.

SECTION

SECTION II.

*Of the evacuations, depofitions, and erup-
tions obferved in Acute Difeafes; and
of the Prognoftic to be derived from
them.*

§ CXLIV. TO treat Acute Difeafes in
a fuitable manner, and
to be enabled to form a Prognoftic in
fuch cafes, the phyfician muft neceffarily be acquainted with every thing that
relates to their fpontaneous folution.

§ CXLV. To prepare and bring about
fuch or fuch an evacuation, or depofition, or eruption, are the means which

we

we every day fee nature exerting herfelf
to effect, in the cure of difeafes.

§ CXLVI. These fpontaneous folutions
of Acute Difeafes, are obferved both in
thofe patients who are left wholly to nature, and in thofe who are placed under
the care of phyficians.

§ CXLVII. The mode of treatment
may, as we fhall hereafter obferve,
(§ CCCLXXXIII & feq.) have fome influence on thefe fpontaneous folutions, fo
as to render them more or lefs frequent,
according to the remedies that are employed.

§ CXLVIII. When a fpontaneous folution is performed quickly, it is called
crifis; when it takes place gradually
and by degrees, it retains the name of
folution.

§ CXLIX. The adjective, *critical*;
when employed to characterize an evacuation, or eruption, or depofition, im-
plies

plies it to be falutary, and contribu-
ting to the happy termination of the
difeafe. The adjective, *fymptomatic*, is
employed in a different fenfe, and being
added to an evacuation, &c. conftantly
means, that it contributes neither to cure
nor even to mitigate the difeafe.

§ CL. An Acute Difeafe is faid to have
attained a ftate of coction, when it pre-
fents the figns which evince the difpofition of nature, to bring about the falutary
evacuation which is to terminate the difeafe. (See § CLXVIII, CXC, CCLXXIX,
CCLXXXII, CCLXXXIV.)

§ CLI. These preliminary ideas will
be fufficient for the underftanding of
what is to follow. This important matter, will be more fully treated, and with
greater propriety, when we have pointed
out the favourable, or unfavourable
figns, that may be derived from carefully
attending to evacuations and depofitions,
and eruptions, according to their various
qualities,

qualities, and the different circumſtances that accompany them.

§ CLII. A DISRELISH for all ſolid and liquid food ; languor and nauſea at the ſtomach ; general weakneſs ; pain and heavineſs at the fore part of the head ; vertigo ; cardialgia ; trembling of the lips ; and ſalivation ; theſe are the uſual fore-runners of vomiting.

§ CLIII. IF, at the beginning, or during the courſe of an Acute Diſeaſe, the patient vomits up a bilious, mucous matter, and feels himſelf relieved by it : ſuch a vomiting is a good omen, and contributes to moderate the diſeaſe.

§ CLIV. WHEN a vomiting is inceſſantly tormenting the patient, without affording him any relief ; we may conclude it to be ſymptomatic. It marks the violence, and, very often, the danger of the diſeaſe.

§ CLV.

§ CLV. The relief which does, or does not, follow, is in vomiting, as in every other evacuation, eruption, &c. in the course of a fever, the most certain mark by which we can determine the good or unfavourable Prognostic that is to be drawn from it.

§ CLVI. This truth (§ CLV.) is equally applicable to the vomiting, we excite by an emetic.

§ CLVII. A critical vomiting is announced by the signs (§ CLII.) we lately mentioned, combined with the signs of coction. (§ CLXVIII, CXC, CCLXXIX, CCLXXXII, CCLXXXIV.)

§ CLVIII. It is, by no means, usual to see an acute fever terminate by vomiting.

§ CLIX. When at the onset of an acute fever, the patient is tormented by an obstinate, laborious, and symptomatic vomiting; we have reason to expect a

grievous

grievous and dangerous difeafe. The
fmall pox, however, is an exception to
this obfervation. The degree of danger
in that difeafe, not feeming to depend
on the obftinate or laborious vomiting
that accompanies it in the beginning.

§ CLX. If, during the courfe of an acute
fever, the patient is tormented with frequent naufea, and without effect, the
fymptom announces danger. *Hip.* 134.

§ CLXI. Every fymptomatic vomiting
announces danger; but if the patient vomits pure bile, of a deep yellow colour,
the Prognoftic will be ftill more unfavourable. *Hip.* 135.

§ CLXII. There is even more danger
when the patient vomits a green coloured
bile. *Hip.* 131.

§ CLXIII. A vomiting of atrabilis in
Acute Difeafes, announces a fpeedy death.
(* 17.) *Hip.* 131, 132.

§ CLXIV. The Prognoſtics we have juſt now deſcribed, (§ clxi, & ſeq.) are equally applicable to acute fevers, that are the conſequence of wounds. *Hip.* 133.

§ CLXV. The vomiting of black blood, whether it be liquid or grumous, altho' it be accompanied with a bad pulſe, and ſigns of the greateſt debility, does not, however, in acute fevers, afford ſo unfavourable a Prognoſtic, as the vomiting of atrabilis. (§ clxii.)

§ CLXVI. If the humours voided by vomiting, depoſit a minced matter, a kind of grounds ⁎ : we may be aſſured that the Iliac vomiting, as well acute as chronic, has taken place, and this is conſtantly accompanied with great danger. (⁎ 18.)

§ CLXVII. The ſtools, do in the courſe of an Acute Diſeaſe, afford ſigns

---

⁎ The Author's expreſſion, is, " *Si les humeurs rendues par le vomiſſement, depoſent une matiere hachée, une eſpece de marc.*"

which

which are of importance to be known, becaufe they contribute much to the forming a juft Prognoftic. The young phyfician cannot be too early in getting rid of that embarraffment which he may feel in afking to infpect thefe evacuations. The good of humanity is the object of medical fcience, and gives dignity to things, which, in vulgar eyes feem abject and contemptible.

§ CLVIII. It is of advantage in Acute Difeafes, when the ftools are like the natural ones, in their confiftence and other qualities. *Hip.* 137. If, from being liquid, they become of a firmer confiftence, the change is a favourable one. It is a fign of coction that announces the tendency of the difeafe towards a cure. *Hip.* 140.

§ CLXIX. Borborygmata, elevation of the abdomen, fenfation of weight about the loins, a foft, unequal, and fometimes an intermitting pulfe, are the figns which ufually precede diarrhoea, and this, if

K 2

preceded

preceded by the figns of coction, we may
hope will be critical.

§ CLXX. If a diarrhœa comes on in
the early days of an acute fever, which
began its attack with the ufual forerunners
of a dangerous difeafe, (§ ccxciv.) it
would be to prove our inexperience, to
fuppofe, that at fuch a period of the difeafe, this flux can be critical. In truth,
it concurs with the other fymptoms, to
denote, on the contrary, that the difeafe
will be more grievous and dangerous.
Hip. 148.

§ CLXXI. This flux to be critical, muft
be copious.

§ CLXXII. T h e ftools in a critical
diarrhœa, are ufually of a yellowifh
complexion, approaching, more or lefs, to
a brown colour. *Hip.* 140, 141.

§ CLXXIII. The improved practice of
the moderns, feems by a well-timed ufe
of laxative medicines, to render this
kind

kind of crifis lefs frequent than it was with the ancients.

§ CLXXIV. THE diarrhoea that comes on in an acute fever, is often of ufe, tho' it is not perfectly critical. The quality (§ CLXXII.) of the ftools, but above all, the relief the patient feels from them, will render the Prognoftic, more or lefs, favourable.

§ CLXXV. WHEN the diarrhoea is purely fymptomatical, it is to be arranged amongft the unfavourable figns.

§ CLXXVI. THE ferous, copious and fymptomatic diarrhoea, is familiar to malignant fevers, and announces danger.

§ CLXXVII. THE danger of this kind of diarrhoea, is in proportion as the patient is weakened, by the copioufnefs and frequency of the evacuations.

§ CLXXVIII. SUCH a diarrhoea happening to a woman after delivery, is very alarming;

alarming; efpecially if it comes on during the firſt days of her lying-in.

§ CLXXIX. When the ſtools are of the colour of white clay, we may ſuſpect worms.

§ CLXXX. If the patient voids worms, it is better for them to come away dead, and at the cloſe of the diſeaſe, when the ſymptoms ſeem to be on the decline, than alive, and at the beginning of the fever.

§ CLXXXI. Liquid, ſymptomatic ſtools, reſembling the yellow of an egg, in colour, announce danger. If the ſtools are liquid, and of a green colour, they are ſtill more dangerous.

§ CLXXXII. Atrabilious ſtools, or in other words, liquid, dark coloured, livid, or black evacuations, announce the approach of death, as do thoſe which have a cadaverous ſmell.

§ CLXXXIII

§ CLXXXIII. Stools of black, clotted blood, are sometimes the natural consequence of a violent hemorrhage at the nose, when the patient has swallowed much of the blood.

§ CLXXXIV. Similar stools are likewise to be expected when the patient has vomited up much blood.

§ CLXXXV. Dark coloured bloody stools, whether they be liquid or in clots, sometimes take place, likewise, in acute fevers, without any previous hemorrhage at the nose, or vomiting of blood.

§ CLXXXVI. Notwithstanding the extreme weakness of the pulse, and of the system in general; and notwithstanding the great change in the patient's physiognomy, (§ xxv.) which usually accompany these stools, they are not, however, by any means so dangerous, as those which abound with atrabilis. The patient even escapes, in general, if he is well treated, and they seem, on certain occasions,

occafions, to be in fome meafure critical.
(＊ 19.)

§ CLXXXVII. Dysenteric ftools appearing in the courfe of an acute fever,
are to be confidered as of a falutary or
unfavourable tendency, according as they
relieve the patient, or are merely fymptomatic.

§ CLXXXVIII. When a fuppreffed
diarrhoea is followed by tumefaction of
the abdomen, and by increafed weaknefs
and naufea; we may be affured that the
ftate of the patient requires a return of
the flux.

§ CLXXXIX. This fame obfervation
is equally applicable to the diarrhoea, we
may have occafion to notice in chronic
diforders. *Hip*. 154.

§ CXC. It is of ufe in Acute Difeafes,
for the urine to afford figns of coction,
that is, that it be natural as to colour and
confiftence. It is a good fign when the
urine

urine, gradually arrives at, and remains in this ſtate of coction, as we may then hope, that the diſeaſe will be ſoon, and happily terminated. *Hip.* 156, & ſeq.

§ CXCI. We cannot depend on the coction of the urine in the beginning of a fever, unleſs it affords all the ſigns of an Ephemera.

§ CXCII. Nor can we derive a favourable Prognoſtic from urine, which alternately affords marks of coction, and crudity. This variation in the ſtate of the urine, may lead us to conclude, that the diſeaſe is not near its termination.

§ CXCIII. We ſometimes obſerve, in the courſe of malignant fevers, and even ſometimes in other caſes, a little before death, that in the midſt of the moſt grievous ſymptoms, the patient voids urine that is perfectly natural.

§ CXCIV. The phyſician ſhould, therefore, be informed of theſe exceptions.

L

(§ CXCI, CXCII, CXCIII.) They afford us this reflection, that he who founds his Prognostic, wholly on the state of the urine, will be liable to be deceived. We are not to conclude, however, on this account, that the inspection of the urine, is altogether useless, on these occasions.

§ CXCV. The urine, which, from being transparent, when first voided, becomes at length turbid, and deposits a thick, white, uniform sediment, announces the solution of the disease, and is truly critical.

§ CXCVI. This kind of spontaneous solution of Acute Diseases, is usually affected without difficulty. It is not accompanied with any alarming symptom, nor does it merit the name of crisis, if we take that word in its exact sense. (§ CCCLV.)

§ CXCVII.

§ CXCVII. The ſediment (§ cxcv.) is, in general, ſlightly tinctured with red.

§ CXCVIII. Clear, and colourleſs urine, leads to ſuſpect that the diſorder is not likely to terminate ſoon.

§ CXCIX. Urine of this ſort, is ſtill more unfavourable, if it happens in children, whoſe urine is, when in health, uſually leſs limpid than that of adults, and eſpecially of delicate and hyſterical women.

§ CC. Turbid urine, that affords no ſediment, is likewiſe an unfavourable ſymptom.

§ CCI. The ſame thing may be ſaid of ardent urine, which is the more alarming, in proportion as it is of a higher red colour, and in ſmaller quantity.

§ CCII. Ardent urine, that is of a dark brown, or black colour, whether it affords

L 2

a

a fediment, or not, is an unfavourable
fign.

§ CCIII. Galen, Duretus, and many
other authors, affure us, that urine of this
fort, is much lefs unfavourable in women, whofe lochia, or catamenia are fuppreffed.

§ CCIV. Every change in thofe qualities of the urine, (§ cxcviii. & feq.)
towards the period of coction (§ cxc.)
is of ufe: on the other hand it is an unfavourable fign, when the urine, from
being crude, becomes clear, or turbid,
like mare's urine (*Jumentewfe*), ardent, &c.

§ CCV. We are to be careful not to
confound the farinaceous, branny fediment, with the critical depofition (§ cxcv.
cxcvii.) The former being an unfavourable fign.

§ CCVI. In malignant fevers, and other
Acute Difeafes, that partake of their
nature,

nature, a piffing of blood, is a dangerous fymptom.

§ CCVII. Experience proves, that the
retention of urine, which happens in an
Acute Difeafe, is not fo dangerous a
fymptom, as one would be tempted to
fuppofe from bare reafoning.

§ CCVIII. It proves even more than
this; we know that fuch a retention,
fometimes, tho' rarely, ferves as a compleat crifis in fuch difeafes. (* 20.)

§ CCIX. If, during the courfe of an
Acute Difeafe, there comes on a copious,
general, and reeking fweat, by which
the patient feels himfelf relieved; it may
be confidered as ufeful, and as affording
a good fign. It mitigates, and often, being entirely critical, terminates the difeafe. *Hip.* 171, 172, 177.

§ CCX. A speedy, and complete crifis
by fweat, is often *immediately* preceded
by

by that kind of fhivering, called *rigor.*
Hip. 178. (21.)

§ CCXI. The moiſture, and ſupple-
neſs of the ſkin, joined to a ſoft, yielding, open, and undulating pulſe, and the
other ſigns of coction, give us room to
expect a ſweat of ſome kind, which will
either ſimply mitigate the diſeaſe, or be
critical and deciſive.

§ CCXII. Much of the Prognoſtic here,
will depend on the particular temperament of the patient. If his former diſeaſes have uſually terminated by ſweat,
we may, with more certainty, expect it
in this.

§ CCXIII. The ſweat, which terminates the paroxyſms of an intermitting
fever, or the exacerbations of a continued
fever, ſimply announces the end of the
fit, but without operating on the Prognoſtic.

§ CCXIV.

§ CCXIV. THE sweat may be useful even in the first day, in an ephemera, or in catarrh; but we are not to consider it as critical, in the first days of an acute, or malignant fever.

§ CCXV. A PURELY symptomatic sweat, is to be considered as an unfavourable sign. *Hip.* 173.

§ CCXVI. THE sweat, which appears only on the forehead, the face, or the neck, while the rest of the body continues dry, is to be considered as symptomatic. It announces, in Acute Diseases, a degree of danger, which can be determined only by considering the other symptoms of the disease.

§ CCXVII. COLD sweats, either partial or general ones, (§ ccxvi.) when preceded and accompanied by other of the most alarming symptoms, announce a speedy death. *Hip.* 174, 175, 176, 179.

§ CCXVIII.

§ CCXVIII. Every body knows that parts of the body expofed to the air, while fweating, eafily become cold; we ought, therefore, to learn to diftinguifh the coldnefs of thefe fweats, from thofe fatal ones which precede death, and which are always accompanied by other figns of danger. For want of attention to this, the inexperienced phyfician will be liable to fall into the moft abfurd error in his Prognoftic.

§ CCXIX. The fweat, altho' it be warm, and general, and copious, is fometimes, not lefs certainly the fign of death. When this is the cafe, however, it is accompanied by exceffive weaknefs, the *facies hippocratrica,* anxiety, and in a word, with the moft dangerous fymptoms. This kind of fweat, is fometimes of a vifcid confiftence.

§ CCXX. Acute Difeafes, are fometimes terminated by an hemorrhage from the nofe. *Hip.* 127.

§ CCXXI.

§ CCXXI. THIS kind of crifis, is peculiar to patients who are between the ages
of fourteen and five and thirty years.
Hip. 180.

§ CCXXII. THE practice of the moderns feems to render critical hemorrhages from the nofe, lefs frequent than
they were with the ancients.

§ CCXXIII. THE youth of the patient,
his particular difpofition to bleeding at
the nofe, a rebounding pulfe, flufhing of
the face, heavinefs, tinnitus aurium, and
itching at the noftrils, are the principal
circumftances, which, when combined
with the figns of coction, (§ CLXVIII, CXC,
CCLXXIX, CCLXXX11, CCLXXXIV.) give us
reafon to expect that the difeafe will foon
be determined by a crifis of this kind.
Hip. 180, 181, 182.

§ CCXXIV. IF the face is remarkably
more florid on one fide than on the other,
we may prefume that the blood will flow
from the noftril on that fide.

M   § CCXXV.

§ CCXXV. This kind of crisis is often preceded by obstinate watchfulness, redness of the eyes, phrenitic delirium, violent pains of the head, and other alarming symptoms.

§ CCXXVI. The hemorrhage from the nose, which procures no relief, is a most dangerous symptom. *Hip.* 184.

§ CCXXVII. If it happens in the course of an Acute Disease, that the patient voids only a few drops of blood from the nose; such an hemorrhage cannot be critical. It must be arranged amongst the dangerous symptoms, especially in subjects of a riper or advanced age. *Hip.* 183.

§ CCXXVIII. In young persons, if this symptom is accompanied, or followed by the signs we before mentioned, (§ ccxxiii.) it concurs with them in announcing a critical hemorrhage.

§ CCXXIX. In female patients, a copious, and premature discharge of the
catamenia,

catamenia, fometimes fupplies the place of hemorrhage from the nofe, by quickly terminating Acute Difeafes.

§ CCXXX. IF the period of menftruation happens, during the courfe of an acute fever, it is ufeful for it to take place in due order, and in the ufual quantity.

§ CCXXXI. A LOSS of blood that is merely fymptomatic, affords only an unfavourable fign.

§ CCXXXII. PISSING of blood, and copious hemopthyfis, happen rarely but in malignant fevers, and particularly in the worft kind of fmall pox. Thefe hemorrhages, ufually announce death.

§ CCXXXIII. SWELLINGS of the parotid glands, are equally obferved in peftilential and malignant fevers. Buboes in the groin, or axilla, or neck, belong more particularly to peftilential fevers. *Hip.* 186, 188.

§ CCXXXIV.

§ CCXXXIV. A BUBO is of ufe, when its appearance fenfibly relieves the patient. It is critical, when it caufes the fever, and all the other formidable fymptoms that attended it to ceafe. *Hip.* 187. In either of thefe cafes, a fpeedy fuppuration is to be wifhed for. *Hip.* 191.

§ CCXXXV. WHAT we have faid of the bubo, may be equally applied to fwellings of the parotid glands.

§ CCXXXVI. THE fudden difappearance of either of thefe, is followed by death, unlefs they are fpeedily replaced by fome fimilar tumour, or by a critical evacuation. *Hip.* 186, 192.

§ CCXXXVII. THE gradual refolution of thefe tumours, is not attended with the fame danger.

§ CCXXXVIII. SYMPTOMATIC buboes, or fwellings of the parotid glands, announce a fpeedy death. *Hip.* 187.

§ CCXXXIX.

§ CCXXXIX. In time of the plague, the bubo which appears in a man, who is in other respects healthy, is to be considered as a preservative; it proves that this man having been affected, nature has happily deposited the pestilential virus in this tumour, without giving time, as it were, to the disease to unfold itself.

§ CCXL. The carbuncle is a frequent symptom in pestilential fevers. We sometimes observe it, likewise in the malignant fevers of Lower Languedoc, Provence, &c.

§ CCXLI. When the eruption of a carbuncle occasions the cessation of the fever, and of the formidable symptoms that accompanied it; and when the gangrene which characterizes this tumour, soon stops, the carbuncle may be considered as critical, and likely to terminate disease.

§ CCXLII.

§ CCXLII BUT if nature does not ſtop the progreſs of the gangrene ; and if ſuitable remedies are ineffectually employed this purpoſe : if the fever continues, and the pulſe becomes more and more frequent, ſmall, ſoft, and weak ; the carbuncle is then to be conſidered as purely ſymptomatical, and can afford only the moſt dangerous Prognoſtic.

§ CCXLIII. BLACK livid eruptions, are to be arranged amongſt the moſt pernicious ſymptoms in the ſmall pox, and eruptive fevers.

§ CCXLIV. WHEN, during the courſe of an acute fever, the integuments of the poſteriors, become gangrenous ; we may be aſſured of the violence and danger of the diſeaſe.

§ CCXLV. THE Prognoſtic will be ſtill more unfavourable, if the tendency to mortification appears every day to advance more rapidly.

§ CCXLVI.

§ CCXLVI. But, if a laudable fuppuration takes place, and a feparation of the found, from the mortified parts, we may judge favourably of the event.

§ CCXLVII. Violent pains in the legs and feet; and the eruption of *vibices*, or fpots, refembling the marks of ftripes; together with a dark, livid complexion of thofe parts, are amongft the figns of approaching death.

§ CCXLVIII. It fometimes happens, however, that thefe fymptoms are the effect of a falutary and critical gangrene: this may be difcovered, by obferving the fymptoms of the difeafe difappear, in proportion as the gangrene becomes eftablifhed. *Hip.* 206.

§ CCXLIX. Acute fevers, which run out to a great length, without affording any alarming figns, as ufually terminate by fome inflammatory depofition or abfcefs. *Hip.* 193, 194, 195.

§ CCL.

§ CCL. IF an acute fever changes its character, and terminating in a flow fever, excites cough, oppreffion, fixed pain in fome part of the breaft; and an inability of fleeping but on one fide, without adding to all thefe fymptoms; thefe figns give room to fufpect, that the acute fever is terminated by a depofition on the lungs. (§ CCCCLXXIV, & feq.)

§ CCLI. IT is well for the patient's countenance to become extenuated, in proportion to the violence, and length of the difeafe; but if, during the fix or eight firft days of an acute fever, his face appears to be unchanged, or even to become fuller than it was in health; we may confider this as a fymptom peculiar to malignant fevers. *Hip.* 198.

§ CCLII. THE fwelling of the face at the clofe of an acute fever, is ufually falutary and critical. This fort of crifis is peculiar to malignant fevers.

§ CCLIII.

§ CCLIII. IF, in the course of an acute-fever, the patient is attacked with eryfipelas, either on the face or legs, fuch an eruption is ufually of ufe, and fometimes is completely critical.

§ CCLIV. BUT if the eryfipelas affords no relief, it is to be confidered as fymptomatical only, and of courfe, as an unfavourable fign.

§ CCLV. THE fort of eruptive fever, which, from its principal fymptom, has been named eryfipelas of the face, is in general, free from danger.

§ CCLVI IF, at the beginning of fuch a fever, we find the patient extremely languid, and complaining of frequent naufea, and faintnefs, with a quick, fmall, foft, weak, irregular pulfe; thefe fymptoms ought not to alarm us. The marks of beginning eryfipelas, which we obferve on fome part of the face, and ufually firft about the nofe, give us reafon, not to fear much from thefe fymptoms.

N   Vomiting,

Vomiting, and the complete eruption of the eryfipelas ufually terminate them.

§ CCLVII. If, when the eryfipelas is complete, the fever ceafes, the diforder is fhort, and occafions but little inconvenience.

§ CCLVIII. But if the fever continues after the eruption, the difeafe will be longer, and more troublefome.

§ CCLIX. If the acute fever, which accompanies eryfipelas of the face, affords during its courfe, the fymptoms of a malignant fever, the difeafe is then truly dangerous. Thefe cafes, however, are rare.

§ CCLX. The metaftafis, or tranfpofition of gouty, inflammatory, eryfipelatous, or purulent humours, are favourable, whenever they pafs from within, outwards; and are on the other hand alarming, and dangerous, whenever they take a contrary direction. *Hip.* 199, & feq.
§ CCLXI.

§ CCLXI. If retrocedent gout produces apoplexy, angina, or inflammation of the breaft or lower belly; a fpeedy death is ufually the refult, unlefs we can fucceed in calling back the gout to the feet.

§ CCLXII. In the rheumatifm, the difeafe fometimes affects the lungs, and excites cough, dyfpnoea, and hemopthyfis; but with much lefs dangerous fymptoms than are produced by retrocedent gout. (22.)

§ CCLXIII. If, at the beginning of an acute fever, the pains in the thighs and legs, fuddenly ceafe, and are fucceeded by phrenitic delirium, and pain in the fide; we have every thing to fear from fo unfavourable a change. *Hip.* 200.

§ CCLXIV. If, from an error of nature, or the rafh and improper application of repellent medicines, eryfipelas of the face, fuddenly difappears, and is

N 2   fucceeded

fucceeded by delirium, and lethargy; we may fufpect the greateft danger.

§ CCLXV. WHEN the copious fuppu-ration of a wound is fuddenly ftopped; we have to fear left the pus, being ab-forbed, and carried into the circulation, depofit itfelf on fome of the vifcera, and occafion the death of the patient.

§ CCLXVI. NATURE, fometimes, puts an end to acute fevers, by throwing out innumerable apthæ, and by a copious falivation.

§ CCLXVII. PETECHIAL fevers, which are often produced by the infected air of fhips, and prifons, and hofpitals, ufu-ally afford the fymptoms that are com-mon in malignant fevers; we are, there-fore, carefully to appreciate thefe fymp-toms, becaufe it is on thefe we are to found our Prognoftic, and not on the eruption which is peculiar to them, and which appears to be in no way critical. (* 23.)

§ CCLXVIII.

§ CCLXVIII. THE eruption of purple fpots, is obferved in peftilential and malignant fevers, and in fome kinds of fmall pox. (*24.) (§ DLXXX, & feq.)

§ CCLXIX. THESE fpots appear on every part of the body, except the face. When they are few in number, they appear chiefly on the neck, and forepart of the breaft.

§ CCLXX. THIS eruption is a moft unfavourable omen. The more numerous, and large, and deep coloured the fpots are, the more certain is death.

§ CCLXXI. LIVID, violet fpots, if any fuch appear in the courfe of a malignant fever, announce a fpeedy, and certain death. *Hip.* 204.

§ CCLXXII. THE *vibices* we have before mentioned, likewife afford a fimilar Prognoftic. It often happens that thefe and livid fpots, do not appear until the

agony

agony of death, or after the patient is dead.

§ CCLXXIII. There is another kind of eruption, a rednefs of the fkin, which, fometimes, tho' rarely, occurs in continued fevers, but without being alarming.

§ CCLXXIV. This fort of eruption, which the French call *porcelaine*, is merely the effect of indigeftion, and is foon diffipated. (* 25.)

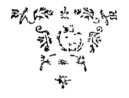

SECTION

SECTION III.

§ CCLXXV. WHEN the patient's tongue, at the beginning of a fever is covered with a thick, whitiſh cruſt, more or leſs inclining to a yellowiſh colour; we may ſuſpect that the diſeaſe will be an acute, continued fever, either mild or dangerous. We very ſeldom obſerve this appearance of the tongue in the ephemera, or in catarrhal, or even intermitting fevers.

§ CCLXXVI. So long as this cruſt continues to become thicker, 'and dryer, and

and of a deeper colour; we may conclude, that the difeafe ftill goes on aug-
menting.

§ CCLXXVII. It is only in the moft
dangerous acute fevers, that this cruft is
found to affume a red, brown, or dark
colour, and then the tongue becomes
dry, and rough to the touch, and the
foreteeth are covered with a dry blackifh
cruft.

§ CCLXXVIII. But, when we obferve
that the edge of the tongue begins to
moiften, and that this cruft gradually di-
minifhes, while the mouth becomes hu-
mid, and the gums refume their natural
vermilion; we may conclude thefe to
be favourable figns. They prove that
the faliva is duly fecreted, that the tran-
fpiration is reftored to the whole infide
of the mouth, and that the diforder has
attained a ftate of coction.

§ CCLXXIX. It is likewife a favourable fign, when the eyes of the patient,
from

from being dull and obfcure, refume
their natural clearnefs. And when his
countenance, from being weak and languifhing, becomes firm, and penetrating.
All this will lead us to hope that the
difeafe will foon happily terminate. *Hip.*
216.

§ CCLXXX. If the patient breathes
with his mouth open, we cannot form
any opinion from the drynefs of his
tongue.

§ CCLXXXI. If his little effort to put
out his tongue to the phyfician, is fufficient to excite a tremor in it; we **may**
argue a weaknefs which belongs **only to**
the moft dangerous malignant fevers.

§ CCLXXXII. If the paffage of the
noftrils, after having been clofed during
the courfe of the difeafe, becomes moif-
tened, fo that the patient is able **to**
breathe, with eafe, through the nofe,
this fign concurs with the other figns,
(§ CCLXXVIII, CCLXXIX.) to denote the
ftate

ſtate of coction, and to announce, that
the favourable termination of the diſeaſe
is at hand.

§ CCLXXXIII. Dryness, and aſperity
of the ſkin, are to be conſidered as unfavourable ſigns, nor ſo long as they continue, can we ſuppoſe the diſeaſe to be
near its end.

§ CCLXXXIV. But, if the ſkin, from
being dry and rough, becomes ſoft and
moiſt as in its natural ſtate, this will be
a good ſign, and will argue, that the
diſeaſe is about to terminate.

§ CCLXXXV. The ſigns of coction
(§ CLXVIII, CXC, CCLXXVIII, CCLXXIX,
CCLXXXII, CCLXXXIV.) give us room to
expect ſpeedy and a favourable termination of the diſeaſe.

§ CCLXXXVI. Whenever an evacuation, or an eruption, or a depoſition of
matter, ſeem ſalutary by their qualities,
and above all by the remarkable diminution

nution of the fymptoms, we may expect a cure.

§ CCLXXXVII. The relief which is the effect neither of a falutary eruption, nor depofition, nor evacuation, is faithlefs, and we are not to flatter ourfelves that it will be lafting. *Hip.* 219.

§ CCLXXXVIII. Intermitting fevers, and remittent fevers, which, from the redoubling, or the lengthening out of their paroxyfms, affume the type of continued fevers, are an exception to this rule. (§ cclxxxvii.) The bark, often happily puts a ftop to both thefe without any evacuation.

§ CCLXXXIX. These evacuations, depofitions, and eruptions, when purely fymptomatic, are to be confidered as unfavourable figns. *Hip.* 217, 218.

§ CCXC. When we attempt to irritate or affift nature in Acute Difeafes, by venæfection, emetics, cathartics, leech-

es,

es, finapifms, veficatories, &c. it is well if
thefe means produce the wifhed for relief. If they do not, nor in any way
mitigate the fymptoms, it is an unfavourable fign.

§ CCXCI. If, the patient, at the beginning of an acute fever, complains of
violent pains in the back and loins; we
may expect that the difeafe will be à
a dangerous one. *Hip.* 223.

§ CCXCII. Acute pains in the legs
and thighs, give room for the fame Prognoftic. *Hip.* 225.

§ CCXCIII. If thefe pains fuddenly
ceafe, and are fucceeded by pain in the
fide, or inflammation in any of the vifcera, or delirium, the change is commonly fatal. *Hip. ibid.*

§ CCXCIV. Nausea, difficult and obftinate vomiting, (§ clix.) with cardialgia and anxiety; ferous, or bilious diarrhoea, that is altogether fymptomatic;
(§ cxlv.)

(§ CXLV.) together, with a conftantly
fmall, foft, weak, quick, and often unequal pulfe (§ II.); joined to proftration
of ftrength, (§ XXIII.) and pains, (§ CCXCI,
CCXCII.) are the principal fymptoms,
which, at the beginning of an acute fever,
will give us reafon to expect that it will
be a dangerous one. Peftilential and
malignant fevers, ufually begin in this
way.

§ CCXCV. DEAFNESS, at the beginning
of an acute fever, if added to a fwelling
of the face, (§ CCLI.) contributes to the
certainty of fuch a Prognoftic.

§ CCXCVI. A PHYSICIAN, who in the
firft days of an acute fever, is interrogated concerning its character, fhould reply with prudence and circumfpection,
until its true nature is clearly developed.
Experience will teach him, how neceffary this referve is. They who deviate
from it are frequently obliged to acknow-
ledge themfelves to have been deceived;
or what is ftill worfe, are led, perhaps,

to

to defend their errors, and to excufe them, by means, which are repugnant both to candour and truth.

§ CCXCVII. WHEN an acute fever runs on to the feventh or eighth day, without affording any of the fymptoms which characterize dangerous fevers; we may be affured that the patient will be in no danger.

§ CCXCVIII. IN the courfe of an acute fever, it is often of importance to be able to forefee nearly how long it will laft.

§ CCXCIX. THIS anticipated knowledge of the duration of an acute fever, will be derived in the firft place from its fpecies. We know that the cholera morbus terminates within twenty-four, or thirty-fix hours, and fometimes in lefs time: that in the plague, it is not uncommon to fee patients die within a few hours from the attack, while in others, this cruel difeafe runs out feveral days: that towards the decline of the epidemic, the

difeafe

difeafe is ufually mitigated, and its progrefs becomes lefs rapid : that in other
epidemical fevers, theré is great variety
in their duration : that continued fevers,
and inflammatory fporadic fevers, ufually
terminate within fourteen, or twenty
days, and fometimes fooner, when they
deftroy the patient : that the acute rheumatifm, rarely terminates before the thirtieth day, that it fometimes continues even
to the fixth and feventh week : that the
kind of continued fever, I have defcribed
in another work*, under the name of
the malignant fever, peculiar to young
people, (*fievre maligne des Jeunes gens,*)
runs out to the fiftieth, and even fixtieth
day, when it terminates happily : that
the apoplexy is often inftantaneoufly
mortal, fometimes within a few hours,
a day, or thirty-fix hours; and that, if a
fever follows the attack, it becomes a
true comatofe remittent fever; this fecondary difeafe, ufually continues four-

---

* Memoires fur les fevres aiguês.

teen

teen or twenty days: that the mild and difcreet fmall pox, ufually terminate within ten or eleven days; while the confluent and malignant run out, even to the feventeenth and twentieth day, when they end well.

§ CCC. The more the progrefs of an acute fever is rapid, and the fooner, and more rapidly the fymptoms, of danger begin to appear, the more reafon we have to expect that it will foon terminate either in death or a cure.

§ CCCI. The vulgar adage. " *That which is violent, does not laft long,*" is pretty generally true in fevers.

§ CCCII. When the fever is uniformly violent, the pulfe very quick, ftrong, and elevated, joined to much thirft, and inquietude, and to a burning heat of the fkin; we may reafonably conclude, that the difeafe will be of fhort duration, or at leaft, that it will not continue long in this ftate.

§ CCCIII.

§ CCCIII. But, if during the firſt eight or ten days of an acute fever, which attacks a patient in the flower of his age, we obſerve, that this diſeaſe makes not any ſenſible progreſs, altho' the ſtrength of the patient is beat down, and his pulſe is quick, ſmall, weak, and ſoft, with little heat of the body; we may preſume, that the diſeaſe will be ofthat kind of malignant fever, which is very ſlow in its progreſs, and runs out to the fortieth, and even beyond the fiftieth day, when it terminates in health.

§ CCCIV. In viſiting the firſt patient, the phyſician ſoon becomes acquainted with the character and progreſs, and duration of an epidemic fever.

§ CCCV. Pestilential and malignant fevers, as well epidemic as ſporadic, are fatal in proportion to the rapidity of their progreſs.

§ CCCVI. Intermitting fevers are, in general, tho' not always, free from danger.

P § CCCVII.

§ CCCVII. We should be particularly suspicious of those which are accompanied with coma or syncope. It is observable, however, at the same time, that by means of the Bark, the powers of medicine are more efficacious and decisive in these, than in continued fevers.

§ CCCVIII. In remitting fevers, the Prognostic is to be derived from the symptoms that arise during the exacerbation.

§ CCCIX. If, therefore, the physician neglects to visit his patient at that time, he exposes himself to errors in his Prognostic, which may be injurious to his reputation, and fatal to his patient.

§ CCCX. It is a good sign, when the exacerbation is attended only by a simple increase of fever, and its usual concomitants: such as pain of the head, anxiety, heat, thirst, little sleep, and frequent respiration.

§ CCCXI.

§ CCCXI. If the exacerbation brings with it a flight delirium, oppreffion, and cough; or tumefaction of the abdomen, the cafe is to be confidered as more alarming.

§ CCCXII. But we have every thing to fear, when thefe paroxyfms are attended with faintnefs, or fyncope, or phrenitic delirium; comatofe affection; fpafm; exceffive tumefaction of the abdomen; or fymptoms of pleurify or peripneumony; or of inflammation of any of the abdominal vifcera.

§ CCCXIII. It is of ufe when the pulfe continues free and expanded during the paroxyfm. If it becomes foft, fmall, and unequal, it is an unfavourable fign. We particularly obferve this to happen in malignant, remittent, and comatofe fevers.

§ CCCXIV. The exacerbations, in true continued fevers, are announced by coldnefs of the extremities, or cough, or

great

great thirſt, or increaſed anxiety and head
ach.

§ CCCXV. WHEN each exacerbation of
a remittent fever ſets in with ſhivering;
we may conclude it to be a true intermittent, which, by its paroxyſms being
lengthened out, appears under the form
of a continued fever *.

§ CCCXVI. THESE fevers (§ cccxv.)
are obſerved here, only from about the

---

* To this obſervation of the learned author, it may not be
amiſs to add, that the celebrated Dr Cullen, very properly re-
fers all remittent fevers to the claſs of *intermittents*   See his
Synopſis Noſologiæ Method. and his *Firſt lines of the practice of Phyſic.* Both remittents and intermittens, are, in general, to be tra-
ced to the ſame remote cauſes, and agree in having only one exa
cerbation every four and twenty hours, and, in mutually exchang-
ing types, the remittent fever, frequently becoming a clear and
diſtinct intermittent, and both quotidians and tertians, as well
as quartans, as often, by improper management and other cauſes
reſuming the type of a remittent or continued fever —It was
the experienced M de Haen, who firſt obſerved, that in true
continued fevers, there s an exacerbation twice every four and
twenty hours, and this ſeems to be one of the leading charac-
teriſtics of theſe fevers.

middle

middle of fummer, till the beginning of autumn; when they terminate in a falutary manner, they ufually degenerate into fevers that are evidently intermittent.

§ CCCXVII. If a fever, that began its attack under the form of a tertian, or double tertian, becomes continued, and no longer retains the marks (§ cccxv.) of an intermitting fever; we may reafonably be alarmed, becaufe fuch fevers commonly produce the moft dangerous fymptoms.

§ CCCXVIII. So long as the paroxyfms of a remittent fever, become more and more alarming, either by their duration, or the violence of their fymptoms; we may conclude, that the fever is ftill in a ftate of increafe, and, of courfe, of danger; but if the contrary of this is obferved, our Prognoftic will be a favourable one; and we may confider the fever to be in a declining ftate.

§ CCCXIX

§ CCCXIX. In remitting double tertians, the paroxyfms are ufually of unequal violence and duration; and the Prognoftic is to be derived from the fits, which correfpond with each other, on every third day. It will be liable to be erroneous, if we compare one paroxyfm with that which immediately preceded it. (* 26.)

§ CCCXX. If, at the clofe of an unfavourable remitting fever, (the exacerbations of which, have conftantly gone on increafing, and affording gradually the moft formidable fymptoms) there comes on, as it were, a new paroxyfm, or redoubling of the fever, with an exceffive coldnefs of the extremities; and, if this coldnefs is fo extenfive, that not only the patient's feet, but likewife his legs and thighs, feel like marble, and continue fo two or three hours, and fometimes a much longer time; we have reafon to fear left the patient die in the paroxyfm, to which there is fo alarming a prelude.

§ CCCXXI.

§ CCCXXI. IF, to thefe figns (§ cccxx.) there be added hiccup, and an internal fenfation of burning heat, the Prognoftic will be ftill more certainly fatal.

§ CCCXXII. IF, during the courfe of an acute fever, after the moft alarming fymptoms have prevailed, with bad pulfe, much weaknefs, little heat, and even coldnefs of the extremities, the patient complains of a devouring, burning fenfation within; we may conclude, that death is at hand. (* 17.) *Hip.* 207, 209, 210, 211.

§CCCXXIII. THE Prognoftic to be made with certainty, fhould not be founded on one fign only, but on the whole of what the difeafe has afforded, and continues to exhibit.

§ CCCXXIV. THE fymptoms, which, in the courfe of an acute fever, characterize an affection, more or lefs dangerous, of one or more of the vifcera,

are

are the moſt certain ſigns of imminent danger.

§ CCCXXV. Those which indicate great weakneſs, and a languid and near-ly extinguiſhed circulation, if they ac-company thoſe we have juſt now deſcri-bed, are the moſt invariable marks of approaching death. (§ iv, v, xviii, xix, xx, xxi, xxv, xxvii, xxviii.)

§ CCCXXVI. If an ulcer of long ſtand-ing; or the legs and ſhoulders of the patient excoriated, and ſuppurating from the application of a bliſter; ſuddenly dry up: and, if the application of a veſica-tory excites gangrene, inſtead of inflaming and bliſtering the ſkin, we may expect a ſpeedy death. Theſe ſigns are to be added to thoſe I have already cited, as marks of a languid, and nearly extin-guiſhed circulation.

§ CCCXXVII. We may argue the re-covery of the patient, when he has a
profound

profound and eafy fleep, out of which he wakes fenfibly refrefhed and ftrengthened. When his appetite, and ftrength return by degrees, and in proportion to the violence, and duration of the difeafe he has experienced : and when the difeafe has been terminated by a falutary evacuation, or depofition. (§ CCLXXXVI, CCLXXXVII.)

§ CCCXXVIII. Circumstances contrary to thofe we have now mentioned, will threaten a relapfe.

§ CCCXXIX. The duration of the convalefcent ftate, and the management it exacts, will be proportioned to the violence, &c. of the preceding difeafe. *Hip.* 233.

§ CCCXXX. Pregnant women, attacked with acute fevers, are more liable to fall victims to them, than other fubjects. They are likewife likely to mifcarry during the attack. *Hip.* 234.

Q   § CCCXXXI,

§ CCCXXXI. Loss of blood, long and obstinate diarrhoea, dysentery, and tenesmus, dispose a pregnant woman to miscarry. *Hip.* 235, 236.

§ CCCXXXII. Epileptic convulsions, which precede, accompany, or follow delivery, are, in general, fatal.

§ CCCXXXIII. Of these convulsions, the least fatal ones, are those, which being occasioned by the violence, and duration of the labour, disappear after that is over.

§ CCCXXXIV. A sudden delivery, unaccompanied with pain, is to be suspected; especially, if the patient has before been languishing, or sick, and if the lochia, are of a bad quality, deliveries of this sort, are often followed by the most fatal effects. *Hip.* 238.

§ CCCXXXV. It is a good sign, when a lying-in woman, remains three or four days without fever, and feels no other inconvenience,

inconvenience, than what is incompatible with her fituation, fuch as general weaknefs, &c. and when the lochia flow properly, both as to quality, and quantity, and when, after the third, fourth, or fifth day, the milk fever begins to appear, and then, that the flow of milk takes place.

§ CCCXXXVI. It often happens, in confequence of the irritation of her labour, that the lying-in woman has a little fever, on the firft and fecond day. This, however, will not be alarming, if the lochia flow properly, and the pulfe is free and expanded, and the fkin moift; but above all, if there is no fymptom that threatens any affection of the vifcera.

§ CCCXXXVII. If, in the firft days of a lying-in, and before the milk has appeared, there comes on an acute fever; we have every thing to fear for the life of the patient.

Q 2 § CCCXXXVIII.

§ CCCXXXVIII. If, at this period of lying-in, the patient becomes abfent, or has flight delirium; or ftammers, during a few inftants; if fhe feels, tho' without reafon, as if fhe had received a blow on the back part of her head; fuch fymptoms are not to be confidered as mere vapours. We ought to know, that the patient is, in this cafe, threatened with a depofition of milk on the brain, or with malignant fever.

§ CCCXXXIX. If the patient is attacked with apoplexy, or feels frequent returns of epileptic convulfions, and between thefe, continues in a ftate of lethargy; we may conclude, that the depofition on the brain, has actually taken place. When this happens, the patient, commonly dies, very foon, and fuddenly.

§ CCCXL. If, with fuppreffed lochia, the lying-in woman, has a very fmart fever, pain, hardnefs, and tenfion, about the region of the uterus, and conftant delirium;

lirium: we may conclude, that the uterus is in a flate of inflammation, and this
is, in general, fpeedily followed by
death.

§ CCCXLI. If, during the firft days
after her delivery, the patient is attacked
with horripilatio. and to this there fucceed, fever with head ach; drynefs of
the fkin; diarrhoea; fuppreffed lochia;
acute pains, either in the groin, or iliac
region, or fome other part of the
lower belly; we have to fear, left fome
of the parts there, are become affected
with inflammation. This is a diforder
that is full of danger, and rapid in its
progrefs, efpecially when it affects the
ftomach. *Hip.* 240.

§ CCCXLII. Pleurisy, or peripneumony, coming on about the fame period, are, likewife, marks of great danger.

§ CCCXLIII. But if without any of
thofe figns, (§ cccxxxix, et feq.) the ly-
ing-

ing-in woman is attacked with an acute fever, which begins with vomiting, or a diarrhoea, together with a quick, fmall, foft, and weak pulfe; we know from thefe figns, and thofe which follow afterwards, that fhe has a malignant fever; her fituation renders this cafe particularly dangerous.

§ CCCXLIV. From the fifth or fixth day after delivery, after the milk has begun to flow, until the eighteenth, the patient is liable to thefe inflammatory depofitions of milk, on the vifcera. They very feldom take place, however, except during the firft days of the lying-in.

§ CCCXLV. These depofitions, ufually take place in the cellular texture of the peritonæum, in one of the iliac regions. They excite acute, and obftinate pain, accompanied with fever. When well treated, they ufually terminate in refolution; fometimes, they fuppurate, and bring the patient into danger.

A

A Digreſſion concerning CRISIS, *and* Critical Days.

§ CCCXLVI. THE word *criſis,* is Greek. It may be ſaid, literally, to imply *judgement.*

§ CCCXLVII. THE criſis of an Acute diſeaſe, is, therefore, that operation of nature, which, at a certain period of the fever, produces ſuch a change in the ſtate of the patient, as determines either his death, or his recovery.

§ CCCXLVIII. A CRISIS is ſaid to be ſalutary, when this effort of nature is followed by an evacuation, or depoſi-tion, or eruption ; which alters the ſtate of the patient for the better, and lays the foundation for his cure.

§ CCCXLIX.

§ CCCXLIX. It is ftiled *mortal*, when by producing a contrary effort, it occa-fions death.

§ CCCL. The period of this latter cri fis, is evidently the time, when the dif-eafe produces fome irremediable affec-tion of one or more of the organs effen-tial to life.

§ CCCLI. It often happens, that the patient does not die till two or three days after this mortal crifis.

§ CCCLII. The day of death, is, therefore, the period, at which, the ef-fect of fuch a crifis is confummated. But this day is far from being always the fame as that on which the crifis be-gins to operate.

§ CCCLIII. The word *crifis*, however, is more commonly received in a favour-able fenfe, to imply only the falutary termination of a difeafe.

§ CCCLIV,

§ CCCLIV. We ufually diftinguifh two kinds of falutary crifis; the one of thefe is fudden in its effects, and the other flow, and by degrees.

§ CCCLV. The firft are ufually preceded and accompanied by alarming fymptoms. Thus, while the patient feels the moft fenfible agitation, great heat and fever, together with delirium, his diforder is fuddenly terminated, *judged* as Hippocrates ftiles it, by a copious flow of blood from the nofe.

§ CCCLVI. The fecond kind of falutary crifis, ufually takes place without any apparent aggravation of the fymptoms, at the time. The ufeful evacuations, which are the refult of thefe crifes, often continue for feveral days, and during all this time, the difeafe is gradually difappearing, till at length, it is wholly terminated. Thus, the pleurify, and peripneumony, are commonly terminated by a laudable, free, and copious expectoration, which continues many

R   days,

days, and gradually relieves, and at length cures the patient.

§ CCCLVII. To fpeak correctly, and with precifion, and to avoid, as much as may be, every fource of mifunderftanding, and confufion, Phyficians would do well to apply the word *crifis*, only to the firft of thefe two kinds, and to give to the others, as has been, fometimes, done, that of ＿＿, or folution.

§ CCCLVIII. This diftinction has been, almoft always neglected, and this inaccuracy has introduced errors, and confufion, into the numerous works, we have, on the fubject of crifis.

§ CCCLIX. Acute Difeafes, are, fome-times determined by a fingle evacuation, or depofition. Sometimes two or three evacuations concur to this end, either at the fame time, or one after the other. Sometimes, likewife, a depofition, and one or more falutaty evacuations, concur

at

at the fame time to put an end to the complaint.

§ CCCLX. The crifes, properly fo called, and likewife thofe by folution, are either complete or incomplete. The firft are ufually decifive, and terminate the difeafe; while the incomplete ones, only afford a degree of relief; after which, fome new crifis of the firft or fecond kind, takes place, and puts an end to the complaint.

§ CCCLXI. The crifes, properly fo called, are often immediately preceded by alarming fymptoms. (§ ccxxv.) *Hip.* 241.

§ CCCLXII. The abfence of the fymptoms, which denote a grievous, confirmed, and irremediable affection of fome vifcus; and the prefence of the figns of coction, (§ clxviii, cxc, cclxxviii, cclxxix, cclxxxii, cclxxxiv.) combined with thofe which give us room to expect fuch or fuch a crifis, enliven the hopes

R 2   of

of the phyſician, who has carefully ſtudied nature, and the ſteps ſhe purſues in
the cure of an Acute Diſeaſe.

§ CCCLXIII. WE are able to diſtinguiſh the ſigns which give us reaſon to
expect an hemorrhage from the noſe,
(§ ccxxiii.) or vomiting, (§ clii.) or
diarrhoea, (§ clxix.) or critical ſweats.
(§ ccxxi.)

§ CCCLXIV. BUT there are no ſigns
which announce, with any probability,
that the criſis will be by urine.

§ CCCLXV. NOR, if we expect the firſt
veſtiges of thoſe beginning tumours, are
there any poſitive and probable ſigns of
the approaching eruption of carbuncle,
or bubo, or eryſipelas, or ſwelling of the
parotid glands.

§ CCCLXVI. WE cannot even ſay
with preciſion, whether thoſe tumours
will be ſymptomatic, or critical. This
deciſion can, in my opinion, only be
known

known in the event, at leaſt with reſpect
to buboes, and other abſceſſes; the eryſipelas being, commonly of uſe, and very
often, completely critical.

§ CCCLXVII. There are ſome Acute
Diſeaſes, in which the criſes, properly
ſo called, are more frequent than in
others. In ſome they are unknown.

§ CCCLXVIII. These criſes, are particularly obſerved in peſtilential fevers.

§ CCCLXIX. And in malignant fevers,
which make a rapid progreſs, and likewiſe in continued fevers, of an inflammatory nature.

§ CCCLXX. The cholera morbus, is,
as it were, a diſorder that is wholly critical. This criſis ſeeming to begin with
the complaint itſelf.

§ CCCLXXI. Nature uſually terminates malignant fevers, whoſe progreſs
is ſlow, in the way of ſolution. Thoſe
that

that are more rapid, and inflammatory
fevers, are, likewife, frequently terminated in the fame manner.

§ CCCLXXII. Simple continued fevers, are terminated in the way of folu-
tion˟. The fame thing may be faid of
acute rheumatifm.

§ CCCLXXIII. Of thirty pleurifies, or
peripneumonies, hardly one will be
found, that is fuddenly terminated by
fweat, (§ ccix, cch.) or by hemorrhage
from the nofe. the others will terminate
by a laudable expectoration, by urine,
or ftool, or critical moifture of the
fkin.

§ CCCLXXIV. To cure that kind of
acute continued fever, which is in fact,
only a double tertian, (the paroxyfms being lengthened out, give it the type of a

---

* See the Author's " Memoires fur les fievres aigues."

continued

continued fever,) nature ufually brings it to the form of a regular tertian.

§ CCCLXXV. He who in a malignant intermittent fever, neglecting the ufe of the bark, fhould wait in expectation of a crifis, would be, evidently, an unguarded practitioner, void of any knowledge of the difeafe.

§ CCCLXXVI. Nature cures the fmall pox, by fucceffive crifes. After having effected the firft of thefe, which is the eruption, fhe feems to repofe her-felf. Then follows the fuppurative ftage, to which, when the difeafe is of the con-fluent kind, is added the critical fwell-ing of the hands and feet *, and the fali-vation

---

* Some very ingenious phyficians differ from our author here, and will not allow the fwelling of the face and hands, or the falivation, to be critical, but merely the effect of inflamma-tion, from a greater number of puftules; of this number is, the learned Profeffor Camper, who expreffes himfelf in the follow-ing manner, on the fubject. " Omnes medici, inter quos " Rhafes, Sydenhamus, Meadius, Huxhamus, aliique emi-" nent,

vation, in adults. Neither of thefe, fuddenly terminate the difeafe.

―――――――――――――――

" nent, intumefcentiam faciei, quæ 7, vel 8. die: et manu-
" um, pedumque, quæ 9. vel 10 die poft eruptionem obfer-
" vatur, criticam habuerunt: adeo ut Sydenhamus maximam
" fpem falutis in ea ftatuat: quamquam nonmodo Meadius
" fed et nos fæpiffime viderimus morientes ea ipfa fub condi-
" tione, id eft dum facies maxime tumebat.

" Re igitur exactius examinata arbitrati fumus, hanc intu-
" mefcentiam nullo modo effe criticam; fed proportionatam
" numero puftularum · fuper facie idcirco rariffime tumor ob-
" fervatur in infitione, nifi ultra 50 dentur puftulæ, etiam non
" in manibus ac pedibus. Quorum intumefcentiæ, non quia
" materia critica prius caput, dein inferiora membra occupat,
" fed ideo tardius confpiciuntur, quoniam puftulæ tardius
" in pedibus, quam manibus, ac in facie erumpunt.

" Imminuto igitur numero variolarum intumefcentia illa,
" quam femper coma comitatur, et falivatio, erunt imminu-
" tæ: et quidem adeo, ut omnino nulla intumefcentia, nullus
" foporofus affectus, nulla falivatio nullus manuum, vel pedum
" tumor obfervetur, fi, quemadmodum, in infitione frequenter
" contingit, vel nullæ, vel decem adfummum in facie puftulæ
" dantur.

" Intumefcentiæ hæ igitur non funt criticæ, fed veræ fequelæ
" inflammatioris cutis, et panniculi adipofi; fi vero critica effet
" hæc inflatio, eo major foret intumefcentia, quo minor copia
" puftularum, quod tamen neutiquam obtinet: nam vbi paucæ
" vel nullæ puftulæ, ibi nulla intumefcentia. Idem de faliva-
" tione cenfendum." *De Emolumentis, &c. Infitionis variolarum.*
Pag. 20 *et feq.*

§ CCCLXXVII.

§ CCCLXXVII. Nature does not shew less variety in the spontaneous solution, than in the progress of epidemical diseases, as well as in their symptoms and duration.

§ CCCLXXVIII. Whenever an hemorrhage from the nose terminates an Acute Disease, it is to be considered as a true crisis. It is peculiar to youth, and is more frequent in inflammatory fevers, than in malignant fevers, in which the pulse is small, soft, and weak.

§ CCCLXXIX. The critical vomiting, (§ clvii.) critical swellings of the parotid glands, buboes, carbuncles, (§ccxxxiv, ccxxxv, ccxli.) and likewise critical erysipelas, do all terminate Acute Diseases by a true crisis.

§ CCCLXXX. Crisis, by eruption either of bubo, carbuncle, or swelling of the parotid glands, is peculiar to pestilential and malignant fevers.

S   § CCCLXXXI.

§ CCCLXXXI. Sweating (§ ccix, ccx.) likewife terminates Acute Difeafes by a true crifis. A gentle and long continued moifture of the fkin, terminates them in the way of folution.

§ CCCLXXXII. A similar termination is fometimes the refult of laudable expectoration, difcharges by urine, or ftools, or by fwelling of the face.

§ CCCLXXXIII. The practice firft adopted by Sydenham, feems to render critical hemorrhages from the nofe, lefs frequent now, than they were with the ancients.

§ CCCLXXXIV. The prudent ufe of laxative medicines towards the clofe of Acute Difeafes, does likewife often anticipate the operations of nature. Thefe remedies do, on thefe occafions, feem to determine the evacuation of the matters, which, by the critical efforts of nature, have been previoufly lodged in the primæ viæ.

§ CCCLXXXV.

§ CCCLXXXV. The phyſician is like-wiſe in certain caſes able to aſſiſt, and even determine a critical ſweat. (*28.)

§ CCCLXXXVI. Every day's experi-ence proves to us, that the efforts of na-ture, to bring on an expectoration in cer-tain caſes, may, by the proper or impru-dent uſe of venæſection, and other means, be either aſſiſted, or on the other hand, ſuſpended, and even prevented.

§ CCCLXXXVII. The phyſician ought to be aware of all theſe facts, (cccLIX et ſeq.) whenever he viſits a patient, or em-ploys his thoughts on the criſis. By neg-lecting theſe particulars, we ſhall conti-nue to apply to Acute Diſeaſes in general, certain obſervations, which belong only to a few of that claſs, and thus by con-fuſing the ideas of the young practitioner, our writings, if conducted on ſuch erro-neous principles, would only ſerve to embarraſs him in his practice.

S 2   § CCCLXXXVIII.

§ CCCLXXXVIII. Of the number of days which an Acute Diſeaſe may be liable to laſt, there is not one, on which it may not be liable to terminate, either in a ſalutary or fatal manner. So, that every day may be critical, in whatever ſenſe we accept the word.

§ CCCLXXXIX. But if ſome of theſe days, are more remarkable than others, for being the period of ſuch critical termination, they certainly deſerve to be noticed, and named by way of excellence, *critical* days.

§ CCCXC. The doctrine of Hippocrates on this ſubject, is neither conſtant, nor uniform. If we compare together different parts of his writings, we ſhall find him contradicting himſelf. In his aphoriſms, for example, Sect. iv, xxxvi. he names the third, the fifth, and the ninth, amongſt the critical days; whereas he excludes them from this rank in another part of his aphoriſms, and likewiſe in his books of the Prognoſtics, and of

critical

critical days; in both of which he names only the fourth, the feventh, the eleventh, the fourteenth, &c. *Hip.* 242, & feq.

§ CCCXCI. GALEN feems to have fixed the opinion of Phyficians in general, on this doctrine of Hippocrates. According to Galen, the father of phyfic confidered the fourth, the feventh, the eleventh, the fourteenth, the feventeenth, and the twentieth, as favourable critical days; and to thefe he added the twenty-fourth, the twenty-feventh, the thirtieth, the thirty-fourth, and the fortieth.

§ CCCXCII. ACCORDING to Galen like-wife, the feventh is the moft remarkable of all thefe days, for the frequency and folidity of the crifes, that happen on that day.

§ CCCXCIII. HE is not fo favourable to the fixth day, he even ftiles it the ty-rant of Acute Difeafes, becaufe it is re-markable, he fays, for the number of fatal terminations that happen on it.

§ CCCXCIV.

§ CCCXCIV. The fourth is both a *critical* and an *indicating* day. If the figns of coction appear on the fourth day, they announce a falutary crifis on the feventh. This laft is likewife a day of indication for the eleventh, and this again for the fourteenth. *Hip.* 246.

§ CCCXCV. Such, in a few words, is the doctrine of Galen, and his followers, concerning the critical days, and on this doctrine, we will make the following reflections.

§ CCCXCVI. By a long continued habit of ufing words, the true and precife meaning of which, we have never properly examined, we come very often, at length to adopt the moft abfurd opinions. This feems to have been the cafe with refpect to critical days.

§ CCCXCVII. Acute Difeafes, differing very confiderably from each other, both as to their violence, and duration; the days which will be critical in fome, will

will be far from being fo in others. It would be as abfurd, for example, in the acute rheumatifm to confider the feventh day as critical, when the difeafe may be expected to run out to the thirtieth, or more, as it would be to form expectations from the twenty-fourth, or thirtieth day of a peftilential fever, when a very fmall number of days is likely to terminate the difeafe.

§ CCCXCVIII. We are not, therefore, loofely to fix on any days as being critical to Acute Difeafes in general, becaufe thefe difeafes have no common affinity with each other in this refpect.

§ CCCXCIX. It would be interefting, however, to prove, from careful and attentive obfervation, what is the progrefs, and ordinary duration of each of thefe difeafes, and then to fee whether fuch or fuch an acute fever, has a certain fixed period for its termination.

§ CCCC.

§ CCCC. Such obfervations only, can throw the neceffary light on the difpute concerning critical days. So long as we neglect this, and thus continue to adopt the idea of critical days, in a loofe fenfe, as common to all the different kinds of Acute Difeafes, we are abandoning, as it were, this important part of the hiftory of difeafes, to obfcurity and unanfwerable difficulties.

§ CCCCI. In the eruptive fever, which precedes the eryfipelas of the face, the fecond or third day is frequently critical, becaufe the eruption never removes the fever, and alarming fymptoms, that accompanied it.

§ CCCCII. In the cholera morbus even the firft day is critical.

§ CCCCIII. The plague does not feem to obferve any regular period; that difeafe terminates on the firft, fecond, third, or fourth day; and fometimes later, when

when the diforder is more flow in its progrefs *.

§ CCCCIV. Hippocrates in his *epidem*, lib. i. has faid, that in tertian remitting fevers, the critical days, whether good or bad, are determined by the paroxyfms. So that if the paroxyfms of a fingle, remitting, tertian, or double tertian, happen on even days, the crifis will take place on an even day, and vice verfa.

§ CCCCV. To form a proper Prognoftic, however, in fevers of this fort, I believe it will be of more importance to derive it from the character of the difeafe, the nature of the evacuations, and the ftate of the vifcera, than from the particular type of the diforder, which induces its paroxyfms to happen on even, or odd days.

---

* See the writings of Diemerbroek, and likewife thofe of the Phyficians who defcribed the plague at Marfeilles.

§ CCCCVI.

§ CCCCVI. In inflammations of the breaſt, which terminate favourably by expectoration, the evacuation goes on gradually, and continues many days. It would, therefore, be hard to ſay, in theſe caſes, which of theſe days is critical.

§ CCCCVII. The ſame thing may be ſaid of all Acute Diſeaſes, which terminate by ſolution. If on the eleventh or twelfth day of an Acute Diſeaſe, a gentle moiſture appears on the ſkin, or the urine depoſits a ſediment, and either of theſe ſigns continues two or three days, while the diſeaſe is evidently declining, and at length terminates; which of theſe days ſhall we conſider as the critical one, ſhall it be that which began the criſis, or that on which the diſeaſe terminated?

§ CCCCVIII. In an infinite number of caſes, it would be equally difficult for us to point out the critical day, even when the diſeaſe terminates in death; we have already ſhewn (§ CCCL, CCCLI.) that this fatal criſis, uſually begins one, two,

or

or three days before that period, and is
then only confummated.

§ CCCCIX. The plague, which makes
fo rapid a progrefs, has certainly, with
refpect to critical days, nothing in common with that kind of fporadic malignant fever, which is peculiar to young
people, and feldom terminates before the
thirtieth day, and which fometimes runs
out to the fortieth, and even fiftieth day,
when it ends well.

§ CCCCX. And yet thefe two difeafes
will, to the eye of the attentive obferver,
afford many marks of analogy. They
are both of the fame genus, and the interval which feparates them, is filled up
by fevers, which differ, more or lefs from
each other, by infinite fhades, and gra-
dations, and which have each their particular period.

§ CCCCXI. So that even allowing the
fourth, or the feventh day, to be truly
critical in the plague, it would by no

T 2 means

means follow, that thefe· fame days are more remarkable than every other, in the other kinds of fevers, which altho' of the fame tribe, are, however, very different in their progrefs and duration.

§ CCCCXII. It is therefore evident, that we have long entertained a very abfurd notion, by confidering it as a general principle, "That in Acute Difeafes, " the critical days, fuch as the fourth, the " feventh, the eleventh, the fourteenth, " &c. are to be confidered as particular- " ly deftined to the critical operations of " nature; and therefore, that it is impru- " dent to difturb her at thefe times, by " remedies, which are rather to be ex- " hibited on the intermediate days."

§ CCCCXIII. It will be anfwered, perhaps, by the advocates for critical days, that giving up the idea of them, as common to Acute Difeafes in general, they wifh only to know, whether or not, acute fevers that are rapid in their progrefs, terminate chiefly on the fourth or feventh day,

day, by favourable crifis; and whether
fevers, that are next to thefe in duration,
do not chiefly end on the eleventh or
fourteenth; while others, that are ftill
flower in their progrefs, terminate on the
feventeenth or twentieth, rather than on
other days?

§ CCCCXIV. To this queftion, I am
difpofed to anfwer, that neither my own
reflections, (§ cccxcvii, & feq.) and experience, nor the numerous hiftories of
Acute Difeafes, we meet with in authors,
induce me to believe, that nature affects
any fort of conftancy in terminating thefe
complaints, on the days that have been
named critical. That it is, therefore, a
mark of imprudence and error, to form
our Prognoftic from, or to adopt our method of treatment to, thefe imaginary periods; and that without attending to
them, we fhould found our opinion and
practice wholly on the figns which characterize the difeafe, and indicate the
rapidity, or flownefs of its progrefs, the
ftate of the vifcera, the marks of crudity
and

and coction, and thofe which enable us
to afcertain the ftrength of the patient,
and the critical or fymptomatic evacuations that have taken place, or are likely
to happen. In one word, that we fhould
unite together all the figns that have been
defcribed in this treatife. (* 29.)

§ CCCCXV. The obfervations of Hippocrates, afford fo many examples, repugnant to the doctrine of critical days, that
they alone would be fufficient to authorize the fentiments we have now adopted
concerning them. (˙˙ 29.) See *Profper Alpini de Prefag*. *Lib*. vi. *Cap*. iv.

§ CCCCXVI. I flatter myfelf, that
many of the moft celebrated Phyficians,
now living in Europe, think as I do on
this matter; of thefe, I will content myfelf
with naming Sir John Pringle, who, rejecting the doctrine of critical days, is,
neverthelefs attentive to obferve on every
occafion, the ordinary duration, and particular period of each kind of fever,
and the manner in which it ufually terminates.

minates *. The fpirit of philofophy, which is now fo happily prevalent in medicine, as well as in every other branch of natural hiftory, feems every day to leffen the blind and enthufiaftic refpect our predeceffors paid to the writings of Hippocrates and Galen. We do well, indeed, to profit from, and admire the excellent obfervations they drew from nature; but furely, as men of reafoning, and philofophers, we have a right to difcufs their opinions with freedom, and to reject them whenever they are repugnant to experience and truth.

---

* Obfervations on the difeafes of the army, 7th edit. 8vo. pages 140, 297, 315.

SECTION

SECTION IV.

§ CCCCXVII. THE figns we have already defcribed in the three preceding fections of this work, have the fame Prognoftic fignification in pleurify and peripneumony, as in other acute fevers.

§ CCCCXVIII. But both thefe difeafes have other figns peculiar to themfelves, and which are of confequence to be underftood, if we wifh to know how they will terminate.

§ CCCCXIX. As they occur rarely in infancy, fo are they more dangerous at that age, than in youth, or more advanced life.

§ CCCCXX.

§ CCCCXX. THEY are more frequently fatal, in the robuſt and vigorous, and in thoſe who are addicted to ſtrong liquors, than in other ſubjects. *Hip.* 219.

§ CCCCXXI. THEY are likewiſe very dangerous in aſthmatic patients.

§ CCCCXXII. IN the pleuriſy, it is a good ſign when the pain, affecting only one ſide, is ſupportable, and does not much affect reſpiration.

§ CCCCXXIII. VIOLENT pain in the ſide, denotes a dangerous pleuriſy.

§ CCCCXXIV. BUT, if this pain becomes ſo acute as to render the breathing exceſſively ſhort, and to excite cries and groans in a man, who has fortitude, and is naturally patient of pain, the Prognoſtic will be very unfavourable. Its fatality will be more confirmed, if repeated bleeding affords no relief.

U   § CCCCXXV,

§ CCCCXXV. When the pains, in thefe cafes,, affects the upper parts of the breaft, *Hip.* 254, the back, and mediaftinum, they are much more dangerous than thofe which are lateral, and lower down.

§ CCCCXXVI. If the pain varies, both as to its feat and violence, being, fometimes, very fharp, and then almoft entirely ceafing ; we may fufpect that the patient has worms, either in the ftomach or inteftines.

§ CCCCXXVII. If the matter of expectoration is ftreaked with blood; and the patient feels a pain in fome part of the breaft, which tho' obfcured from time to time by a more acute pain, appears again when that is over; we may conclude the difeafe to be a pleurify complicated with worms.

§ CCCCXXVIII. In circumftances oppofite to thofe we have now defcribed; we may conclude, that without the

exiftence

exiftence of true pleurify, the pain (§ ccccxxvi.) is wholly occafioned by worms; and this fecond cafe is, therefore, much lefs dangerous than the firft.

§ CCCCXXIX. The known character of the reigning difeafes, and the figns we have formerly defcribed, (§ xl, xli.) will enable us to diftinguifh thefe two cafes. (§ ccccxxvii, ccccxxviii.)

§ CCCCXXX. A pain in the fide, that is truly and wholly pleuritic, may likewife change its feat, either by a removal, or by an extenfion of the inflammation: the pain of the newly affected part, by its greater violence, rendering the patient lefs fenfible of the other. *Hip.* 252.

§ CCCCXXXI. In this cafe, which is full of danger, the new pain is fixed and conftant, and does not afford the variety we defcribed in the other cafes. (§ ccccxxvii, ccccxxviii.)

U 2 § CCCCXXXII.

§ CCCCXXXII. If the pain of the side, and difficulty of respiration disappear, and are succeeded by phrenitic delirium, we have reason to fear, that the disease will terminate in death. (*30.) *Hip.* 251, 273.

§ CCCCXXXIII. If the pain of the side, and fever are violent, it is better for them to be so at the beginning: but, if from being moderate at that period, they both become very acute about the sixth day, our Prognostic will be very unfavourable. *Hip.* 253.

§ CCCCXXXIV. If a very acute pain in the side, suddenly ceases, without our being able to attribute this relief to a sweat, or hemorrhage, or any other critical evacuation; and, if at the same time, the other symptoms which distressed the patient, invrease, instead of diminishing. If he becomes cold, has cold sweats, bad pulse, and much change in his physiognomy; we then know, with certainty, that death is at hand.

§ CCCCXXXV.

§ CCCCXXXV. In the pleurify and peripneumony, the difficulty of breathing, is ufually proportioned to the violence of the difeafe.

§ CCCCXXXVI. It is therefore of ufe for the refpiration to be neither very difficult, nor quick, but full; and it will be well, likewife, if the patient complains of no more cough or oppreffion, when lying one fide, than when lying on his back; and that he fleeps in this laft pofture, if he has been accuftomed to it.

§ CCCCXXXVII. In general, the Prognoftic in thefe difeafes will be more unfavourable, in proportion as the refpiration is fhorter, and more laboured and difficult.

§ CCCCXXXVIII. The different degrees of difficult refpiration, cannot be eafily defined; habit and experience, only, can enable the phyfician to diftinguifh them properly.

§ CCCCXXXIX.

§ CCCCXXXIX. Altho' the patient has more cough, and is lefs eafy when lying on one fide, than on the other, we are not, however, to be too hafty in concluding, that he has an abfcefs of the lungs. (§ cccclxxxiv.)

§ CCCCXL. This fymptom (§ ccccxxxix.) appearing at the beginning of a pleurify, or peripneumony, fimply announces that the inflammation affects only one lobe, or one lobe more than the other.

§ CCCCXLI. If, during the courfe of a pleurify, or peripneumony, the patient is fuddenly feized with fo great a difficulty of breathing, as to be obliged to fit upright in his bed, and that even in this fituation, his refpiration is laborious: and if this fymptom has not been preceded by the figns of an abfcefs, (§ cccclxxiv, & feq.) we may prefume, that an effufion has taken place into the cavity of the breaft, and this will be fufficient to announce the approach of death. (* 31.) *Hip.* 255.

§ CCCCXLII.

§ CCCCXLII. If the blood drawn off is fizey, it is well when the buffy coat is not very thick, and when there separates from the congulum, after a convenient time, a sufficient quantity of serum.

§ CCCCXLIII. But if the buff seems to extend thro' almost the whole of the coagulum, and is at the same time transparent like a jelly: if the surface is variegated with livid spots, and if the blood, after being long at rest in the porringer, does not separate into serum, and craffamentum, we may conclude that death is near at hand*; and,

---

* The reader, who is aware of Mr. Hewson's ingenious experiments on the blood, and who knows that the existence of buff often depends merely on the size of the orifice, porringer, &c. will probably object to what the author has advanced here, and will be inclined to think, that the appearance of the blood can afford only a feeble support to the Prognostic in these cases. I had prepared the same objections. The learned author will be found replying to them in his note * 32, at the end of this work.

indeed,

indeed, this sign is always attended with moft alarming fymptoms. (˘ 32.)

§ CCCCXLIV. A soft and expanded pulfe, is in general, a favourable fign in inflammation of the breaft. It ufually precedes, and accompanies the falutary expectoration, which terminates thefe difeafes.

§ CCCCXLV. If the fymptoms become every day more grievous; and the pulfe, from being ftrong, feels empty, (§ v.) or fmall, weak and unequal; this change announces great danger. It is ufually accompanied by the moft fatal fymptoms. (§ iii.)

§ CCCCXLVI. Hardness of the pulfe is by no means effential to pleurify. This fymptom is to be arranged amongft the figns of the Prognoftic in this difeafe. (* 33.)

§ CCCCXLVII. This fymptom is an unfavourable fign, when it continues
long,

long, and with a certain degree of ſtea-
dineſs.

§ CCCCXLVIII. So long as this hardneſs of the pulſe continues, we are not
to expect any ſalutary and deciſive expectoration.

§CCCCXLIX. If, when the other ſymptoms do not threaten death, this hardneſs
of the pulſe continues till the eleventh
day; we may then very properly ſuſpect,
that the diſeaſe will turn to ſuppuration
and abſceſs.

§ CCCCL. When the pulſe, even on
the firſt days of inflammation of the
breaſt is very frequent, ſmall, weak, ſoft,
and often irregular; the diſeaſe may be
conſidered as participating of the nature
of malignant fevers. (§ 11.) In theſe there
is much more danger than in the others,
and blood-letting, inſtead of being uſeful,
is often very pernicious. They turn to
gangrene, much more frequently, than
pleuriſy that is purely inflammatory.

X   § CCCCLI.

§ CCCCLI. One of the moſt favourable ſigns that can happen in theſe caſes, is, when the pulſe diminiſhes in frequency, but becomes more expanded, ſtrong and regular.

§ CCCCLII. As pleuriſy and peripneumony, when they end favourably, generally terminate in a laudable and copious expectoration, it is right to be acquainted with the different qualities of the matter that is ſpit up, and how much either of theſe will influence the Prognoſtic.

§ CCCCLIII. When expectoration is wholly deficient in either of theſe diſeaſes, they are extremely dangerous. *Hip.* 256. And altho' when this is the caſe, the ſymptoms do not announce death; we may reaſonably fear that ſuppuration and abſceſs will be the reſult.

§ CCCCLIV. If the matter that is expectorated, has neither colour nor conſiſtence; and is altogether watery, and frothy, like the ſaliva, and at the
fame

fame time affords no relief to the patient, the Prognoftic will be unfavourable. (§ CCCCLIII.) *Hip.* 261.

§ CCCCLV. WE are not to be alarmed when the matter that is expectorated in the beginning of a pleurify or peripneumony, is ftreaked with blood.

§ CCCCLVI. IT is indeed a good fign, when the expectoration begins on the firft days of the difeafe, to eftablifh itfelf in this manner. (§ CCCCXLV.) *Hip.* 265, 267. It is likewife a good omen, when at this period, the patient expectorates without much difficulty, while the matter of expectoration is of a firmer confiftence, and more vifcid than faliva, and fomewhat ftreaked with blood; and likewife, when between the fourth, and the feventh, or eighth day, this appearance of blood is effaced, and the matter that is fpit up, becomes more infpiffated, till at length the patient, every time he coughs, brings up with great facility, a quantity of matter, of a thickifh con-

X 2

fiftence,

fiftence, and of a uniform, darkifh, white colour, approaching, more or lefs, to yellow, or red.

§ CCCCLVII. The relief it affords the patient, will enable us to judge of its efficacy. *Hip.* 271.

§ CCCCLVIII. When it is only after the repeated efforts of an almoft dry cough, that the patient is able to force up, as it were, a little matter, the expectoration of which, affords no relief to the patient; we may conclude, from fo unfavourable a fign, that the cure of the difeafe is as yet very diftant.

§ CCCCLIX. But if the patient feeming to have his lungs fo filled with matter, as to be unable, notwithftanding all his efforts, to fpit it up; and if, after having coughed and expectorated, we diftinguifh by the particular noife he makes in breathing, that a quantity of matter is ftill adhering to the Bronchiæ: we

we have every thing to fear from fo unfavourable a fituation. *Hip.* 264.

CCCCLX. If the fpitting is wholly
of blood in the beginning of a pleurify or
peripneumony, we may expect that the
difeafe will be dangerous. *Hip.* 268. If
fuch an appearance takes place in a more
advanced ftage of the difeafe, it will be
ftill more dangerous.

§ CCCCLXI. A bilious fpitting, that
is, of a tranfparent, gliftening, yellow
matter, is a bad fign. *Hip.* 260.

§ CCCCLXII. That which is of a leek
green, is ftill more dangerous. *Hip.*
262.

§ CCCCLXIII. A spitting of brown,
livid, and black matter, announces, in
general, certain death. *Hip.* 263.

§ CCCCLXIV. If, during the courfe
of a pleurify, or peripneumony, a purulent expectoration gradually takes place,
we

we may attribute it to a fuperficial ulceration of the membrane that lines the Bronchiæ.

§ CCCCLXV. This fort of purulent expectoration is not very copious; whereas, that which is occafioned by the burfting of an abfcefs, (§ D, DI.) comes on fuddenly, and is very copious at the beginning.

§ CCCCLXVI. The expectorations we have defcribed, (§cccclxiv.) occur chiefly in certain cafes. (§ ccccliii, ccccliv, cccclviii, cccclxi.) Pleurifies and peripneumonies that begin with a violent and obftinate vomiting, are ftill liable to afford fuch an expectoration, during their courfe (* 34.) There are other cafes, however, (§ cccclv, et feq.) in which we are not to expect it.

§ CCCCLXVII. The Prognoftic in this cafe, (§cccclxiv,cccclxv.)is to be founded, not on the purulent nature of the expectoration,

expectoration, fo much as on the whole of the fymptoms collected together.

§ CCCCLXVIII. If the expectoration goes on with eafe, if it relieves and vifibly mitigates the fymptoms, we have reafon to expect that the difeafe will be foon, and happily terminated.

§ CCCCLXIX. If, even in the beginning of peripneumony, to great difficulty of breathing, a kind of perturbation (*bouillonment,*) within the breaft, violent fever, and very pliant pulfe, there be joined a copious expectoration of a purulent matter; however alarming thefe fymptoms may be, yet, are we not to defpair of a cure. Experience feems to prove, that peripneumonies of this fort are not commonly mortal. *Hip.* 272.

§ CCCCLXX. If, amidft the moft alarming fymptoms, there comes on a fhivering, which is immediately fucceeded by a very copious and univerfal fweat, which evidently relieves the patient:

this

this fweat is falutary. It terminates the difeafe by a crifis, properly fo called. (§ ccx, cccliv, ccclv.)

§ CCCCLXXI. A moisture of the fkin long continued, and which relieves; as likewife, falutary ftools; (§ clxxii.) critical urine that depofits fediment, (§ cxcv.) all tend to announce a fpeedy and happy termination of the difeafe.

§ CCCCLXXII. If, during the courfe of a pleurify, on the fudden ceffation of all the fymptoms of that difeafe, there comes on a retention of urine; this new difeafe may ferve as a crifis to the firft. Such a crifis, tho' rare, has, however, fometimes happened.

§ CCCCLXXIII. When an inflammation of the breaft runs on to the fourteenth day, without the patient's appearing to be advancing towards a cure, either from the deficiency of a laudable expectoration, or of fome other falutary evacuation; and yet, at the fame time,
the

the fymptoms are not fuch as indicate the difeafe to be mortal ; we have reafon to think that it will end in abfcefs, fuppofing that it is not already formed. *Hip.* 274, 275.

§ CCCCLXXIV. If the fever changes its type, and affuming that of a fuppurative fever, becomes remittent, each of its paroxyfms beginning by a fhivering; we can hardly doubt, but that the difeafe is actually going on to fuppuration. *Hip.* 276, 277, 278, 279.

§ CCCCLXXV. The regular, or irregular returns of thefe paroxyfms, will not alter the diagnoftic. (§ ccccLxxi.) (35.)

§ CCCCLXXVI. The fhiverings with which fuppurative fevers ufually announce themfelves, are commonly much more violent at the beginning, than when they have lafted fome time.

Y   §CCCCLXXVII.

§ CCCCLXXVII. The violence of thefe fhiverings, and the regularity with which they return, are liable to deceive the inexperienced phyfician, and lead him to miftake thefe fuppurative fevers, for fimple remitting, or intermitting fevers.

§ CCCCLXXVIII. The diagnoftic figns of abfcefs, (§ ccccLxxiii, ccccLxxiv.) are confirmed by the following.

§ CCCCLXXIX. The patient is no fooner afleep, whether it be night or day, than he falls into copious fweats, which weaken him, inftead of affording him relief. *Hip.* 280, 282.

§ CCCCLXXX. If pleurify is fucceeded by abfcefs, and the pain ftill keeps the fame feat, it becomes a dull, heavy pain, inftead of being acute, and pungent as it was before this change. *Hip.* 276, 287.

§ CCCCLXXXI. The cough continues, but is of no ufe. It is dry, and affords

only

only a matter fimilar to faliva. *Hip.* 282.

§ CCCCLXXXII. Sometimes the cough raifes a difagreeable odour to the noftrils. This is fometimes fenfible even to the affiftants.

§ CCCCLXXXIII. This fymptom, whenever it occurs, adds to the fatality of the Prognoftic in this cafe, the abfcefs itfelf being fufficiently baneful.

§ CCCCLXXXIV. The cough, oppreffion, and heavy pain in the fide, affect the patient more, when he lies on one fide, than on the other. *Hip.* 281.

§ CCCCLXXXV. The feat of the abfcefs is ufually, tho' not always, on the fide oppofite to that which the patient complains moft of when he lies on it.

§ CCCCLXXXVI. The blood, (fuppofing that the patient requires bleeding,) will be found fizey.

§ CCCCLXXXVII.

§ CCCCLXXXVII. THE fwelling of the feet. *Hip.* 282. and of the hands, and eye lids; together with diarrhoea, or dyfentery. *Hip.* 280, 283; and likewife an unequal and intermitting pulfe, are all fo many figns of abfcefs in the breaft.

§ CCCCLXXXVIII. IF to thefe figns, (§ ccccLXXIII. et feq.) there be added, a troublefome and manifeft pulfation within the breaft, we are not to be too eafily perfuaded that it is an aneurifm.

§ CCCCLXXXIX. AN abfcefs of the lungs, fituated fo as to receive the impreffion of the heart's motion, or of the great arteries, will fometimes occafion a falfe appearance of aneurifm. (* 36.)

§ CCCCXC. IF to the other figns of abfcefs in the breaft, there be joined other formidable fymptoms, fuch as great cough and oppreffion, bad pulfe, violent fever, and great change in the countenance,

nance, &c. we have reason to fear, that the patient will die speedily, and before nature can be able to give vent to the matter contained in the abscess.

§ CCCCXCI. If the symptoms that ac·company it, are not violent; if the patient's breathing is not disturbed; if the pain, and the cough, and the fever are moderate, and the urine and stools as in a natural state; and if at the same time, the patient gets rest at night, the Prognostic will be more favourable. *Hip.* 286. We may venture to say, that the danger will be deferred till after the bursting of the abscess..

§ CCCCXCII. The physician will do well, however, to inform the assistants, that whenever that happens, the patient may, perhaps, die suddenly; either by the pus being discharged at once into the cavity of the breast, and thus occasioning a fatal syncope; or by flowing into the Bronchiæ, and thus suffocating the patient.

§ CCCCXCIII.

§ CCCCXCIII. It is impoffible to fay with precifion, how long a time will pafs between the formation of the abfcefs, and its burfting.

§ CCCCXCIV. The more rapid the difeafe feems to be in its progrefs, and the greater the cough and oppreffion are ; and likewife, the fever, and the heat of the body; the fooner may we expect the abfcefs to difcharge itfelf. *Hip.* 289.

§ CCCCXCV. An abfcefs of the breaft feldom opens fooner than twelve or fifteen days after it has begun to form ; nor later than thirty. *Hip.* 288, 289.

§ CCCCXCVI. The fever, cough, and oppreffion, do fometimes, tho' not always, increafe a little before the rupture of the abfcefs, and give us reafon to fufpect, that this will foon happen. *Hip,* 290.

§ CCCCXCVII.

§ CCCCXCVII. If the increaſed cough affords ſtreaks of blood with the matter that is ſpit up, or a diſagreeable odour, (§ ccccLxxxii,) we may venture to be-lievc, that the abſceſs is about to rupture, and that the diſcharge will be into the Bronchiæ.

§ CCCCXCVIII. If a patient, who has all the ſymptoms of an abſceſs in the breaſt, voids a urine which depoſits a co-pious and purulent ſediment, or is ſeized with diarrhoea, and that either of theſe occaſions the fever, and the other ſigns of abſceſs to ceaſe; we may ſuppoſe, that by a ſalutary effort of nature, the pus is abſorbed, and after being carried through the circulation, is evacuated through theſe outlets.

§ CCCCXCIX. This termination is a very favourable one, but it rarely happens.

§ D. If the abſceſs burſts on the ſide of the Bronchiæ, it is well if this happens
when

when the patient is awake ; becaufe then
there will be lefs danger of his being
fuffocated.

§ DI. In this cafe, we may form a favourable opinion of the event of the
difeafe ; if, at the beginning, the purulent expectoration is eafy, copious, and
of a good quality ; and likewife, if this
difcharge mitigates the fever, and after
having continued feveral days in abundance, at length gradually becomes lefs
and lefs. *Hip.* 291.

§ DII. In circumftances oppofed to
thofe we have now defcribed, we may
expect to fee the patient die confumptive. The Prognoftic will be a doubtful
one, if the ftate of the patient affords at
once, both good and bad figns. *Hip,*
292, 293, 295, 296.

§ DIII. If, before the burfting of the
abfcefs, there appears a tumour in any
external part of the breaft ; we may conclude, that the matter is making its way
towards

towards that part, and that we shall soon perceive a fluctuation, and this, whether the tumour appears inflamed or only white and œdematous.

§ DIV. If, in the mean time, there comes on a copious expectoration of purulent matter, and the tumour disappears; we may conclude, that the abscess has discharged itself into the Bronchiæ.

§ DV. If, on the other hand, this tumour affords signs of evident fluctuation, it will be prudent to open it: and if, by the operation, there is discharged a laudable pus, and that this discharge soon mitigates the fever and cough, and restores the patient to his appetite and sleep; we have every reason to hope that the disorder will terminate well. *Hip.* 298.

§ DVI. When the abscess is opened, if the pus that issues from it is sanious, fœtid, and of a bad colour; and if, with these unpromising qualities of the pus, the slow fever continues; we may con-

Z   clude,

clude, that the patient will die confumptive.

§ DVII. When an abfcefs, either of the lungs or pleura, burfts and difcharges its contents into the cavity of the thorax, the patient ufually experiences a faintnefs, and fometimes a complete fyncope, in the very moment of the difcharge. *Hip.* 297. Then he feels a flight relief, but only for a fhort time, for the difficulty of breathing foon returns, and gradually increafes, till he is obliged to be conftantly in an erect, or fitting pofture ; and at the fame time he complains of a preffure like a belt, about the region of the diaphragm.

§ DVIII. The feat of the pain, whether of the pungent pain, during the courfe of the inflammatory fever, or of the dull, heavy pain, that takes place after the abfcefs is formed, indicates the fide of the breaft, on which we are to expect the difcharge.

§ DIX.

§ DIX. The patient's inability to lie on the oppofite fide, without adding much to the cough and oppreffion, confirms this diagnoftic. *Hip.* 301.

§ DX. We may likewife, on thefe occafions, obferve a fenfible difference in the two fides of the breaft, that in which the difcharge has taken place, appearing to be larger than the other. *Hip.* 301.

§ DXI. This inequality will be more remarkable at the pofterior, than at the anterior part of the breaft.

§ DXII. This laft fign, (§ dx.) however, is obfervable only when the difcharge is very confiderable.

§ DXIII. Surgery alone can afford any relief to the patient in this fituation.

§ DXIV. When the operation of the Empiema has been performed, the good or bad quality of the pus, *Hip.* 298, 299, together with the ceffation, or continu-

ance

ance of the fever, and other fymptoms,
are to guide us in our Prognoftic. Even
in the moft favourable circumftances;
however, it would be imprudent to affure
the cure of fo dangerous a complaint,
till we fee it almoft completed.

§ DXV. Abscess of the lungs, is not
always the refult of pleurify, or peripneumony. It is fometimes a primary
affection, and of itfelf conftitutes the
difeafe.

§ DXVI. Such an abfcefs announces
itfelf by a pain in the breaft, more or
lefs acute; a dry, and frequent cough;
difficulty of breathing; inability to lie
but on one fide; and by a fever, which
from its firft attack, affumes the character of a fuppurative fever, (* 37.) fometimes the pulfe is unequal and intermitting.

§ DXVII. The Prognoftic in this cafe,
will not be different from the other, and
is to be derived from the figns we have

just

juſt now mentioned. (§ ccccxc, ccccxci, ccccxcii.)

§ DXVIII. It now and then happens, that an abſceſs forms in the breaſt, without giving any ſigns of its approach. The patient does not even feel himſelf affected till the period of its diſcharge. This ſort of abſceſs has been properly called purulent vomica.

§ DXIX. The moment the vomica burſts, the pus ſometimes flows into the Bronchiæ, ſo ſuddenly, and in ſo great a quantity, as to ſuffocate the patient inſtantaneouſly.

§ DXX. If he eſcapes, however, and expectorates a great quantity of purulent matter, the Prognoſtic, (§ d, di.) will be the ſame as in the abſceſs that follows pleuriſy or peripneumony.

§ DXXI. The lymphatic, as well as the purulent vomica, does, likewiſe, not manifeſt itſelf till the moment it burſts.

§ DXXII.

§ DXXII. The patient being then seized with a continual and suffocating cough, expectorates a frothy, lymphatic matter, and in great abundance.

§ DXXIII. The fever is soon added to this, and if it continues, we have reason to fear that a purulent expectoration will be confirmed, and that the patient will die consumptive.

§ DXXIV. It sometimes, tho' rarely, happens, that the patient coughs up the lymphatic vomica included in its cyst *, and resembling a small egg deprived of its shell; this is followed by a very copious expectoration of a frothy, lymphatic matter.

---

* What the author calls lymphatic vomica, may perhaps be more properly stiled an Hydatid. There is in the second volume of the Med. Transactions, a curious account of Hydatids, discharged by coughing. It would be superfluous to relate it here, as that work is, or ought to be, in the hands of every practitioner.

§ DXXV.

§ DXXV. The only difference be-tween thefe two cafes, is, that in the former, the vomica burfts; whereas in the latter, it is voided whole.

§ DXXVI. It is likely that the lym-phatic vomica, fometimes fuffocates the patient inftantaneofly. (* 38.)

§ DXXVII. The angina, which is feat-ed in the larynx, and affects the voice of the patient, is the moft alarming. It ufually carries off the patient, the third, or fourth day, and fometimes fooner. *Hip*. 313.

§ DXXVIII. This fort of angina is very happily, exceedingly rare, efpeci-ally with adults. Children are the moft fubject to it.

§ DXXIX. The angina which is feated in the tonfils, and neighbouring parts, only affects the deglutition, and is feldom fa-tal when purely inflammatory.

§ DXXX.

§ DXXX. Sometimes it becomes dangerous, when in such a degree, as wholly to prevent the patient from swallowing.

§ DXXXI. The frequent and copious spitting of a viscid matter, usually relieves the patient, and operates as a sort of crisis to this disease.

§ DXXXII. If one of the inflamed tonsils suppurates, the spontaneous or artificial opening of such an abscess, together with the purulent spitting soon dissipate the fever, and other symptoms.

§ DXXXIII. If the inflammation of the throat is so extensive as to occasion a hard and considerable external swelling, which includes one of the parotids, and the submaxillary glands and muscles, on the same side; and this tumour should suppurate, the patient will run a risk of suffocation, by the sudden bursting of the abscess, if this happens internally.

§ DXXXIV.

§ DXXXIV. Altho' the angina ſhould affect only the deglutition, yet if, from the beginning, the patient feels his ſtrength much weakened, and has a quick, ſoft, weak, and unequal pulſe, we diſtinguiſh that he has the ulcerated ſore throat; a very dangerous diſeaſe.

§ DXXXV. The ſloughs, which ſoon appear on the tumid parts within the mouth, and the infectious breath of the patient, confirm this diagnoſtic.

§ DXXXVI. If, in the courſe of this diſeaſe, the gangrenous inflammation extends to the larynx, and the patient's voice becomes ſhrill, we may deſpair of being able to ſave him.

§ DXXXVII. If peripneumony is added to this complaint, the Prognoſtic will be ſtill more dangerous; and, altho' the patient ſhould not immediately periſh, he will probably die hectic, from the effects of the diſeaſe. *Hip.* 304.

§ DXXXVIII. It is in the flower of their age, between the ages of fifteen and thirty-fix, that men are the moft fubject to hemopthyfis. *Hip.* 305.

§ DXXXIX. It is feldom mortal of itfelf. (* 39.) It is particularly alarming, however, on account of the pulmonary confumption, of which, it often lays the foundation. *Hip.* 306.

§ DXL. But the prudent, and experienced phyfician, will not be fo eafily alarmed by a fpitting of blood, as men are in general. He will know how to difcriminate the cafes that are attended with danger.

§ DXLI. If a patient of a delicate conftitution, and who may be fufpected to inherit a difpofition to phthifis, fpits up in coughing, pure, vermillion coloured and frothy blood, in a certain quantity, as a tea-cup full, for inftance, or more, at once, or at different times ; and, if at the the fame time, there comes on a little

continued

continued remitting fever, the exacerbations of which, are marked by flight fhivering, or merely by a coldnefs of the extremities; all fuch circumftances will be alarming. They will fufficiently indicate the hemopthyfis to be the forerunner of pulmonary confumption; which we know to be an almoft incurable difeafe. *Hip.* 307, 308, 309.

§ DXLII. But if the patient is of a good conftitution, and free from hereditary difpofition to phthifis; or if he coughs up only flight ftreaks of blood, mixed with his faliva, and has no fever, the cafe will threaten no difagreeable confequences.

§ DXLIII. In mixed cafes, the Prognoftic will vary acording as they participate more or lefs of the circumftances defcribed in § DXLI, and of thofe mentioned in § DXLII.

§ DXLIV. The abfence, or the prefence of fever, are the two moft decifive

circumftances

circumftances in the fpitting of blood.
However copious it may be, if there is
no concomitant fever, we may flatter ourfelves, that it will not be followed by
phthifis.

§ DXLV. If, after the ftoppage of hemopthyfis, the pulfe becomes hard, and
continues to be fo, we may expect a
return of the complaint.

§ DXLVI. It is about the age of forty,
or forty-five years, that men become
liable to apoplexy, and likewife to a paralytic diftortion of the mouth, and to
palfy of the tongue. *Hip*. 310.

§ DXLVII. Apoplexy feldom attacks
children, or young perfons; but when
it does, is conftantly fatal.

§ DXLVIII. Men are more fubject to
apoplexy than women.

§ DXLIX. Persons of a corpulent habit, are more liable to this attack than
others.

others ; *Hip.* 311. and efpecially, if they are addicted to indolence, wine, and good living.

§ DL. If a perfon's father or mother died apoplectic, or paralytic, we have reafon to fear, that he will likewife be fubject to the fame complaints, when advanced in life.

§ DLI. When a man has experienced an attack of palfy or apoplexy, we may confider him as having a pre-difpofition to thefe difeafes, and may, therefore, expect that he will, one day or other, fall a victim to apoplexy, or to comatofe fever.

§ DLII. If an adult, or one who is advanced in years, complains of a fixed pain in any part of his head; we may confider him as being threatened with apoplexy or palfy. (* 40.)

§ DLIII. Numbness, and a pricking fenfation in the limbs ; frequent vertigo;
sudden

fudden lofs of memory; momentary abfence, do likewife, at that time of life, feem
to threaten the fame difeafes. *Hip.*
312, 313.

§ DLIV. IF a man, who is more than
fifty years of age, has an hemorrhage
at the nofe, it is likely he will be afterwards attacked with apoplexy.

§ DLV. VIOLENT apoplexy is fatal.
Even in the flighteft degree, it is dangerous; *Hip.* 315, and altho' the patient
fhould not die, it is to be feared he will
remain paralytic.

§ DLVI. COMPLETE infenfibility; ftertor; *Hip.* 316; and inability to fwallow,
are the characteriftics of violent apoplexy, which leave us no hopes of a cure.
(*41.)

§ DLVII. IT is a good fign, when a
patient in apoplexy does not fnore, that
he is able to fwallow whatever we put
into his mouth, and that when pinched, or
pricked,

pricked, he fhews himfelf, by his motions, to be not wholly infenfible of pain. It will likewife be a favourable fign, if fever comes on, and by its continuance removes all the fymptoms of coma. The acute fever that takes place in thefe cafes, is ufually a comatofe remitting fever; the Prognoftic, which may be derived from what we formerly faid. (§ cvi. & feq.)

§ DLVIII. But if, on the appearance and continuance of the fever, the fymptoms of apoplexy increafe inftead of diminifhing, we have reafon to fear that the patient will die.

§ DLIX. If a patient, who has been previoufly weakened by a chronic difeafe, is attacked with apoplexy, his death is fpeedy and certain.

§ DLX. If we pinch, or prick the legs of a patient in a fit of apoplexy, and he draws up one, and not the other of them, the latter will be paralytic. The fame

fame obfervation holds good as to his arms.

§ DLXI. When, in the apoplexy, or in its ufual fucceffion, the hemiplegia, which is commonly accompanied in the beginning, with acute, remitting, coma-tofe fever, the patient, in fwallowing, is attacked with violent cough ; we know that this fymptom is characteriftic of a paralytic affection of the oefophagus, and therefore renders the Prognoftic more unfavourable.

§ DLXII. The fatality of the Prognoftic, however, on thefe occafions, will be pro-portioned to the degree of this fymptom. If the patient has only a flight cough, or does not cough every time he fwallows, the difeafe does not threaten death ; but it will give us reafon to forefee, that the palfy will be obftinate, and difficult to remove.

§ DLXIII. If the oefophagus is fo much affected, that all the liquor the patient

attempts

attempts to swallow passes into the tra-
chea, and excites a rattling noise, together with a sense of suffocation, we may
expect soon to see him die.

§ DLXIV. When a paralytic patient
has convulsive motions, death is certainly at hand.

---

§ DLXV. The Prognostic in small pox
is not to be founded on the violence of
the fever, or other symptoms previous to
the eruption, unless, as very rarely happens, they are in so great a degree, as
to threaten death before this event can
take place. The most gentle, and the
most acute, eruptive fevers, are indiscri-
minat.ly followed by distinct or confluent small pox.

§ DLXVI. It is of use, however, when
the eruption takes place on the third or

fourth

fourth day after the attack of fever, and
when it proceeds rapidly, fo that in twenty-four, or thirty-fix, or forty-eight hours,
it be compleat: that the number of puftules be inconfiderable, and that no new
ones make their appearance after that period: that the belly and the breaft be
free or nearly free from them, and that
the fever ceafe as foon as the eruption is
over: that the puftules be of a rofe colour, firm and elevated: that they increafe rapidly in fize, and begin to fuppurate about the feventh or eighth day
of the difeafe: that this fuppuration be
laudable, and that it be compleated within three or four days, without any other inconvenience than what is infeparable from
pain occafioned by the fuppuration: that
at the height of the fuppuration, each puf-
tule be furrounded at its bafe, by a rofe
coloured circle: that if there be any fever during the fuppurative procefs, it be
moderate: that during the prelude, and
the eruption, the belly be open, and the
ftools natural: that the patient be bound
during

during the fuppuration *: that each puf-
tule in the face, when compleatly fuppu-
rated, change into a yellow cruft, which
afterwards becomes brown: that the puftules in other parts of the body inftead
of drying away, burft and difcharge their
contents. Such is the progrefs of the
fmall pox, when it is of the mild and
difcreet kind.

§ DLXVII. If the eruption appears on
the fecond day, we may expect a dangerous fort of fmall pox; but more fo,
if it breaks out on the firft day, and efpecially if there appears, even at the beginning, an exceffive quantity of puftules
on the face; for this conftitutes the mili-

---

* The author feems to fall into a miftake here; furely in
every ftage of the fmall pox, an open belly will be preferable
to coftivenefs. It might agree with the old doct.ine of coction,
to wifh to fee the patient bound, while the matter was fuppu-
rating, but we now know that this can only add fuel to the difeafe, by promoting the abforption of putrid matter from the inteftines It is, therefore, of the greateft confequence, both in
the diftinct, and confluent fmall pox, that the body be kept
gently open during the whole courfe of the difeafe.

ary

ary fmall pox, which ufually carries off
the patient in a few days.

§ DLXVIII. Three or four puftules
are, indeed, fufficient to characterize the
difeafe, but not to determine the term of
the eruption, which is to be dated from
the time we firft faw puftules making
their appearance.

§ DLXIX. The more flowly the eruption defcends from the face towards the
feet, and the longer it is before it is
compleated, the more dangerous will be
the difeafe.

§ DLXX. All things being nearly e-
qual in other refpects, the danger will be
nearly in proportion to the number of
puftules.

§ DLXXI. If the patient fneezes frequently during the eruption, we may be
affured, that fo long as this fymptom continues, the eruption is not complete.

§ DLXXII.

§ DLXXII. If the mouth, and especially the oesophagus, are lined with pustules, which affect the voice of the patient, and prevent him from swallowing; and if, between the period of the eruption, and that of suppuration, the fever runs high, we may foretel great danger during the latter period.

§ DLXXIII. If, during the period of the eruption, the pustules occasion a violent, and continual itching; this may be considered as one of the signs that announce danger.

§ DLXXIV. This symptom becomes more unfavourable, if in so violent a degree, that the patient tears off the pustules, especially from his face, so that they ulcerate instead of coming to a laudable ulceration.

§ DLXXV. The danger will likewise be proportioned to the slowness, with which the suppuration goes on.

DLXXVI.

§ DLXXVI. THE Chryſtaline ſmall pox is uſually very dangerous.

§ DLXXVII. THE warty kind, in which the puſtules are firm and pale, is likewiſe, in general, fatal to the patient.

§ DLXXVIII. THE miliary ſmall pox (§ DLXVII.) is likewiſe fatal, and quickly terminates in death.

§ DLXXIX. WE have every thing to fear in the event of the ſmall pox, in which the puſtules are flattened at their points, and of a purple colour.

§ DLXXX. PURPLE ſpots, diſperſed between the inteſtines of the puſtules, announce the moſt imminent danger.

§ DLXXXI. IF, amongſt the puſtules, we obſerve ſome that are of a black colour, we may foretel the death of the patient.

§ DLXXXII.

§ DLXXXII. Bleeding of the gums, hemopthyſis, bloody urine, voiding of blood, by vomit or ſtool, and likewiſe bleeding at the noſe, if in great quantity, and merely ſymptomatic, are all fatal. Theſe hemorrhages are particularly obſerved in the ſmall pox. (§ DLXXIX, et ſeq.)

§ DLXXXIII. Atrabilious ſtools, or vomiting, are likewiſe fatal.

§ DLXXXIV. A copious, obſtinate, and ſerous diarrhoea, announces the moſt preſſing danger.

§ DLXXXV. The ſudden depreſſion of the puſtules, is uſually the forerunner of death.

§ DLXXXVI. Delirium, angina, difficulty of breathing, pain in the ſide, and, in a word, any other ſymptoms that denote the influence of the diſeaſe, on any of the viſcera, do, at all times, in the courſe of the ſmall pox, announce the moſt preſſing fing danger; and are altogether fatal, if preceded, and accompanied by a depreffion of the puftules.

§ DLXXXVII. It is of ufe in the confluent fmall pox, for the face to fwell confiderably, during the fuppurative period, and then, going off gradually, to be fucceeded by a fimilar fwelling of the hands and feet; and for the patient, if an adult, to have a copious falivation at the fame time.

§ DLXXXVIII. But if the fwelling of the parts I have mentioned, does not take place in due time, or if, when it is once eftablifhed, it fuddenly goes off, and that the patient's countenance, inftead of being animated, is of a pale, or livid colour, we have reafon to fear, that death is at hand; a fudden, and total fuppreffion of the falivation, is attended with fimilar danger.

§ DLXXXIX.

§ DLXXXIX. The fuppuration being completed, it is a favourable fign if the fever, that acompanied it, ceafes at the fame time. If it continues after this period, and more efpecially if it increafes, we may confider the patient, as being not yet out of danger.

§ DXC. Altho'-the difeafe has been mild, and the puftules of the moft diftinct, and favourable kind; yet, when the fuppuration is over, if they dry up in great hafte, without pouring out their pus; we have reafon to fear fome difagreeable fecondary difeafe, fuch as troublefome boils; or apthelmia, that may be fatal to the fight; or an affection of the breaft, and flow fever. The danger, on thefe occafions, will be proportioned to the number of puftules the patient had.

§ DXCI. If we open the puftules before they are perfectly ripe, that is, before the circular inflammation at their bafe, is perfectly effaced, they will be

C c   filled

filled again with matter, and thus we
shall renew the sufferings of the patient.

§ DXCII. The Prognostic, in the mea-
sles, is to be derived, neither from the
quality of the eruption, nor from the
time of its appearance, or retrocession;
but wholly from the symptoms of the
disease, and particularly from those,
which denote the breast to be more or
less affected.

§. DXCIII. It seldom brings the patient into considerable danger, tho' it
often leaves impressions on the breast,
and throat, that are more or less alarming;

-ing; and fometimes it leaves behind it
very obftinate opthalmia *.

---

* However flight the meafles may be in their attack in
Languedoc, it is certain that, in this country, they are very often
a dangerous and fatal difeafe. Morton relates, that in the autumn of 1672, the meafles carried off three hundred perfons
every week —I am aware that a late writer, in the Medical
Obfervations and Inq. has doubted the truth of this, and has been
led, from a zealous admiration of Dr Sydenham, to fufpect that
Morton's was a hear-fay account, but as his defence amounts
only to a fuppofition, it does not feem to overturn the validity
of Morton's affertion.—Dr. Mead relates, that he had feen the
meafles rage with fo much violence in London, as to prove more
fatal than the fmall pox. The meafles are likewife very often
complicated with other difeafes. Sidobre, Macbride, and
others, have feen them combined with fmall pox.—They will
partake of the remitting marfh fever, or of any other prevailing
epidemic, and their danger will thereby be more or lefs increafed —The following account of the Prognofis in the meafles, which is taken from a late differtation on the fubject, will,
I flatter myfelf, not be improperly introduced here. " In
Rubeola, quae alioquin ordinis boni eft, quaedam tamen haud
laetum eventum denunciant Ita tuffis, fi perpetua, crebra &
vehemens eft, fi cum alvo praecipite & inquietudine conjungitur,
haud vacat periculo, in Peripneumoniam, pulmonis fuppurationem, & Phthifin quandoque definens & fic exitium ferens.
Adeoque hoc verum eft, ut non tam a Rubeola quam ab hac
Peripneumonia fymptomatica illam fubfequente, metuendum
fit, diu in ore Medentium fuerit. Certe quo tempore adminif-
tratio per calorem invaluit, hic frequentiffimus Rubeolae finis
non effe non potuit. Sanguinis quoque profufiones malae funt;

C c 2   neque

neque fudores largi, boni. Quafdam quoque notas eruptio dat. Quæ, fi poft quartum aut quintum morbi diem apparet; fi, ante juftum tempus & fubitò, evanefcit, nec mature reftituitur; fi papulas rubere definentes, maculifve purpureis mifceri coeptas, exhibet, etiam fola, magifque, cum quibufdam notis febrilibus mox memorandis, conjuncta, pro certo mala, fæpe perniciofa eft. Poftremo, hæc febrilia, magnus capitis & oculorum dolor, inquietudo magna, delirium & extremorum artuum frigus, etiamque devorandi difficultas, malam morbi naturam, eoque haud bonum finem indicant.

" Contra, ubi illa malæ notæ figna abfunt, ubi neque tuffis gravior eft, neque febris mala, periculi minimum effe folet. Et licet fanguis immodicè profufus mali ominis effe dictus fit, tamen e naribus ejus ftillicidium judicatorium effe, tuffis fublevata, febrifque & alia fymptomata lenita, argumento funt " *Difputatio Med. Inaug. de Rubeola, Auctore,* Samuele Foart Simmons. *Lugd. Bat.* 1776, 4to.

D E

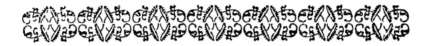

DE PRÆSAGIENDA

in acutis vitâ & morte ægrotantium, selectæ Hippocratis sententiæ.

PRÆFATIO.

§ I. PERÆ pretium mihi facturus Medicus videtur, si ad providentiam sibi comparandam, omne studium adhibeat. Cum namque præsenserit, & prædixerit apud ægrotos, tum præsentia, tum præterita, tum futura, quæque ægri omittunt, exposuerit; res

utique

utique ægrotantium magis agnoſcere cre-
detur: adeò ut majore cum fiduciâ ſeſe
homines medico committere audeant.
Curandi verò rationem optimè molietur,
ſi ex præſentibus affectionibus futura prænoverit. Neque enim fieri poteſt, ut omnes ægroti ſanitatem aſſequantur. Hoc
nempè longè præſtantius foret, quàm
futurorum conſecutionem prænoſcere.
Quandoquidem verò quidam vi morbi
intereunt, priuſquàm Medicum accerſant;
quidam etiam vocato Medico confeſtim,
partim quidem unum diem, partim etiam paulò diutùs vitam trahentes mortui
ſunt, priuſquàm Medicus arte ſuâ ſingu-
lis morbis viriliter ſe opponere poſſit.
Proindè ubi talium affectionum naturam,
quantùm ſcilicet vires corporis ſuperant,
cognoverit; ſimulque & ſi quid divini in
morbis ineſt; hujus quoque providentiam
ediſcere oportet. Hac enim ratione, me-
ritò ſibi admirationem, & boni Medici
exiſtimationem conciliaverit. Qui namque morbo ſuperiores eſſe poſſunt, eos
 utique longè rectiùs conſervaverit, ex
longo antea intervallo ad ſingula conſili-
um

um dirigens; tum etiam morituros, ubi
prænoverit, & prædixerit, extra culpam,
pofitus erit. *Prænot.* 1.

§ II. ATQUE hæc fcribo de morbis acutis & de his qui ab his oriuntur. *Ibid.*
153.

§ III. QUI verò fuperfuturos ex morbo,
& morituros, eofque quibus pluribus diebus, & quibus paucioribus perfeverabit
morbus, rectè prænofcere volet, is intel-
ligentiâ comprehenfam omnium fignorum
doctrinam, æftimare debet, & eorum vires
inter fe collatas ratione expendere, velut
fcriptum eft. *Ibid.* 154.

§ IV. QUIN etiam morborum femper
vulgariter graffantium impetum, & tem-
peftatis conditionem, cito animo conci-
pere oportet. *Ibid.* 155.

§ V. ATQUI quod ad proprias cujufque
rei notas, & reliqua figna attinet, probè
noffe, minimèque ignorare convenit, quod
quovis anno, & quovis anni tempore,
mala

mala malum, & bona bonum denunciant.
Quandoquidem & in Lybiâ, & in Delo,
& in Scythiâ prædicta figna vera effe com-
probantur. *Ibid.* 156.

§ VI. NEQUE verò eft, quod ulliûs
morbi nomen, quod hic adfcriptum non
fit, defideres. Omnes etenim, qui prædictis temporibus judicantur, ex iifdem
fignis cognofces. *Ibid.* 158.

§ VII. MORBORUM acutorum prædictiones non omnino certæ funt nec vitæ
nec interitûs. *Aph.* II. 19.

§ VIII. QUOD fi quis me audiat, is
quám prudentiffimè, & confultiffimè tum
in cæterâ arte, tum in prædictis hujufmodi, fe geret, probè intelligens, qui
prædictionis fucceffum confecutus fit,
apud prudentem ægrum admirationi fore,
qui verò deerraverit, præterquam quod
odio gravabitur, eum ne infaniæ quidem
fufpicionem effugere poffe. *Prædict. Lib.*
II. 6.

Ex

Ex Decubitu.

§ IX. At ægrum à Medico in latus dextrum, aut finiſtrum recumbentem deprehendi oportet, manibuſque & cervice, ac cruribus paulùm reductis, totoque corpore molliter poſito. Hic enim ferè ſani jacentis eſt decubitus. Is autem habetur optimus, qui benevalentium ſimilis eſt. *Prænot.* 8.

§ X. Supinum verò jacere, manibus, cervice, & cruribus porrectis minus bonum. *Ibid.* 9.

§ XI. Quod ſi pronus ad pedes de lecto delabatur, magis formidandum. *Ibid.* 10.

§ XII. Ubi verò pedes nudos, neque admodum calidos habere comperietur, & manus, cervicem, & crura inæqualiter diſperſa, & nuda, malum. Anxietatem enim indicat. *Ibid.* 11.

D d
§ XIII.

§ XIII. Tritæophyæ febres cum jactatione, malignæ. *Coac.* 33.

§ XIV. In acutis exudantes tenuiter &
anxii, malum. *Ibid.* 53.

§ XV. Qui abs re nec ullâ exhaufti
ratione languent, malum. *Ibid.* 54.

Ex Facie.

§ XVI. In morbis autem acutis, in pri-
mis quidem ægroti facies fic in confiderationem adhibenda, fit ne benevalentium, præcipuèque fui ipfius fimilis. Ita
enim optima exiftimanda. Quæ verò ab
eâ plurimùm recedit, graviffimum periculum portendit : qualis fuerit nafus acutus, oculi concavi, collapfa tempora, aures frigidæ & contractæ imifque fuis fibris
inverfæ, cutis circa frontem dura, inten-
ta & reficcata, & totius faciei color ex
viridi pallefcens, aut etiam niger, aut
lividus, aut plumbeus. *Prænot.* 2.

§ XVII.

§ XVII. ITAQUE fi per initia morbi, ejufmodi facies fuerit, neque adhuc ex aliis
fignis conjicere potueris; interrogare convenit, num æger vigilaverit, aut alvus
admodùm liquida fuerit, aut eum inedia
aliqua oppreßerit.   Quod fi quid horum
fateatur, minus formidandum eße exiftimandum. Dijudicantur autem ista, die
ac nocte, fi ex his caufis ejufmodi facies
fuerit.   At fi nihil horum præceßiße dixerit, neque intra dictum tempus ad prif-
tinum ftatum redierit, in propinquo mortem eße fciendum eft. Si verò vetuf-
tiore jam morbo, aut triduo, aut quatri-
duo, talis facies extiterit, inquirenda ea
funt, de quibus antea præcepi. *Ibid.* 3.

§ XVIII. ET reliqua figna, tum ex uni-
verfâ facie, tum ex corpore & oculis, in
confiderationem adhibenda. Si namque
lucem refugiunt, aut illachrymant præter
voluntatem ; aut pervertuntur, aut alter
ex iis minor fit ; aut quæ in iis alba eße
debent, rubefcunt ; aut in iifdem venulæ
livefcunt, aut nigricant ; aut lippientium
oculorum fordes, circa eorum aciem appareant ;

pareant; aut etiam affiduè mobiles, aut tumidi, aut vehementer cavi fuerint; aut eorum afpectus fqualidus, & minimè lucidus; aut totius faciei color immutatus: hæc omnia mala, perniciofaque exiftimanda. *Ibid.* 4.

§ XIX. Quin etiam per fomnum, an ex oculis aliquid fubappareat, fpectare oportet. Ubi namque non commiffis palpebris, ex albo quid fubapparet: id fi neque alvi profluvium, neque medicamentum purgans expreffit, neque ita dormire confueverit æger, pravum eft indicium, & lethale admodum. *Ibid.* 5.

§ XX. Quod fi pervertatur aut corrugetur palpebra, aut livefcat, aut pallefcat, itemque labrum, aut nafus, cum alio aliquo figno, mortem in propinquo effe fciendum eft. *Ibid.* 6. Ubi livores in febre fiunt, propè affore mors fignificatur. *Coac.* 66.

§ XXI.

§ XXI. Lethale quoque, labra refoluta, pendentia, frigida, & exalbida effe. *Prænot.* 7.

§ XXII. Quibus jam morbo fraftis videndi facultas audiendique perit, aut etiam labiorum, palpebrarum, vel narium perverfio cernitur, mors inftat. *Coac.* 72. *eadem ferè Aph.* IV. 49. VII. 73.

Ex Hypochondriis.

§ XXIII. Hypochondrium optimum quidem, quod dolore vacat molle eft & æquale, tum dextrâ, tum finiftrâ parte. *Præn.* 29.

§ XXIV. Quibus hypochondria elevata, murmurantia: dolore lumborum fuperveniente, his alvi humeftantur: nifi flatus èruperint, aut urinæ copia prodierit. *Aph.* IV. 73.

§ XXV.

§ XXV. IN febribus alvo inflatâ, fi flatus liberum exitum non habeat, malum. *Coac.* 44.

§ XXVI. INFLAMMATUM verò, aut dolens, aut intentum, aut inæqualiter affectum, dextrâ parte ad finiftram, hæc omnia animadvertere oportet. *Præn.* 30.

§ XXVII. QUOD fi etiam pulfus infit in hypochondrio; perturbationem aut delirium indicat: verum etiam eorum oculos intueri oportet. Si namque crebro moveantur, infania expectanda eft. *Ibid.* 31.

§ XXVIII. Ex hypochondriorum dolore febres malignæ, quod fi & fopor accefferit peffimum. *Coac.* 31.

§ XXIX. IN febribus acutis convulfiones, & circa vifcera dolores vehementes, malum. *Aph.* IV. 66.

§ XXX.

§ XXX. Ex dolore ventris crudeli cau-
fus lethalis. *Coac.* 130.

§ XXXI. Tumor autem in hypochondrio durus & dolens peffimus quidem,
ubi totem occupat hypochondrium. Sin
verò alteram partem, minore cum periculo finiftram. *Præn.* 32.

§ XXXII. Hujusmodi autem tumores,
circa principia quidem mortem brevi
affore indicant. Quod fi neque intra
vigefimum diem febris quiefcat, neque
tumor fubfidat, ad fuppurationem res vertitur. *Ibid.* 33.

§ XXXIII. His autem primo circuitu
etiam fanguinis è naribus fluxus contingit, valdèque juvat. Verum eos interrogare oportet, num capite doleant, aut
obtufam oculorum aciem fentiant. Quod
fi quid ex his accidat, eo rem tendere
fciendum. In junioribus tamen neque
dum trigefimum quintum annum attin-
gentibus, fanguinis eruptio magis expectanda eft. *Ibid.* 34.

§ XXXIV.

§ XXXIV. Molles autem tumores & doloris expertes, digitifque cedentes, longiores judicationes faciunt, illifque minus graves funt. Quod fi intra dies fexaginta, neque febris ceffet, neque tumor fubfidat, fore fuppurationem hoc loco, & reliquo ventre eodem modo fignificat. *Ibid.* 35.

§ XXXV. Alvi durities cum dolore conjunctâ & cibi faftidio, fi alvo parcè ductâ non expurgetur, in fuppuratum vertetur. *Coac.* 303.

§ XXXVI. Itaque tumores dolentes, duri & magni, periculum mortis intra paucos dies affore fignificant: molles verò & minimè dolentes, quique digito preffi cedunt, illis diuturniores effe folent. *Præn.* 36.

§ XXXVII. Minus verò abfcedunt qui in ventre oriunter tumores, minimè verò qui infra umbilicum; fed ex fuperioribus locis, fanguinis eruptio maximè expectanda eft. *Ibid.* 37.

§ XXXVIII.

§ XXXVIII. Longorum verò omnium in his regionibus tumorum, suppurationes in considerationem adhibendæ. Suppurationum autem quæ indè proveniunt, ea observatio facienda est. Quæ quidem foras vertuntur, optimæ sunt, ubi parvæ sunt, & quam maximè foras feruntur, & in acutum tendunt. *Ibid.* 38.

§ XXXIX. Pessimæ verò quæ magnæ sunt, & latæ, minimèque in mucronem attolluntur. *Ibid.* 39.

§ XL. At quæ intro rumpuntur, optimæ, ubi nihil cum externâ sede communicant, in sese contrahuntur, nullo dolore afficiunt, totaque regio externa unius coloris apparet. *Ibid.* 40.

§ XLI. Hypochondriorum verò dolores, & tumores recentes quidem, & sine inflammatione, murmur solvit in hypochondrio exortum, idque potissimum, si cum stercore urinâ & flatu prodierit. Alioqui ubi ipsum per se transmissum

E e   fuerit,

fuerit, juvat; idque magis fi ad inferiores fedes defcenderit. *Ibid.* 69.

§ XLII. Flatum autem fine fonitu quidem ac crepitu exire, optimum. Præftat tamen cum ftrepitu prodire, quam ifthic revolvi. At qui eo modò prodit, ægrum aliquo dolore vexari, aut delirare indicat, nifi æger fuâ fponte hoc modò ftatum emiferit. *Ibid.* 68.

§ XLIII. Hydropes verò qui ex acutis morbis oriuntur, omnes mali. Nam neque febre liberant, vehementes dolores excitant, & lethales funt. *Ibid.* 42.

§ XLIV. In febribus circa ventrem æftus vehemens, & oris ventriculi dolor, malum. *Aph.* IV. 65.

§ XLV. A cardialagiâ cum torminibus ventris feræ prorumpunt. *Coact.* 285.

En

Ex Respiratione.

§ XLVI. Facilè autem fpirare, valdè magnum ad falutum momentum exiftimandum, cum in omnibus morbis acutis, quibus febris conjuncta eft, tum in his, qui intra dies quadraginta judicantur. *Præn.* 21.

§ XLVII. Spiritus frequens dolorem, aut inflammationem, in locis fepto tranfverfo fuperioribus, indicat. *Ibid.* 18.

§ XLVIII. Qui verò magnus infpiratur, & ex magno intervallo, delirium. *Ibid.* 19.

§ XLIX. At frigidus ex naribus, & ore expiratus, exitialis admodùm jam eft. *Ibid.* 20.

§ L. Lethalis etiam eft æftuofus & fuliginofus: minùs tamen quàm frigidus. Spiritus verò magnus foras efflatus intro parvus, & contra foras parvus intro mag-

nus,

nus, peſſimus eſt, & morti proximus.
Quin etiam tardus, velox, obſcurus, du-
plex intro revocatus; qualis cernitur in
iis qui ſuper inſpirant. *Coac.* 260

§ LI. In febribus, ſpiritus offendens,
malum. Convulſionem enim ſignificat.
Aph. IV. 68. *idem. coac.* 277.

§ LII. In acutis affectionibus, quæ cum
febre fiunt luctuoſæ reſpirationes, malum.
Aph. VI. 54.

§ LIII. Quod ſi dum morbus viget
ægrotus velit reſidere hoc in omnibus
acutis malum, in pulmoniis verò peſſimum. *Præn.* 14.

§ LIV. Si febre detento, tumore non
exiſtente in faucibus, ſuffocatio de repente contingat, lethale eſt. *Aph.* IV. 34.

§ LV. Capitis dolores vehementes, ac
continentes cum febre, aliquo quidem ex
ſignis lethalibus accedente, admodùm exitiales.

itiales. Quod fi fine fignis ejufmodi, dolor vigefimum diem fuperet, & febris dé-
tineat, fanguinis ex naribus eruptionem,
aut alium quemdam abfceffum ad inferiores fedes expectare oportet. Verum
quoad dolor recens fuerit, eodem modò
fanguinis ex naribus eruptionem, aut fuppurationem expectare convenit, cum aliàs, tum fi dolor circa tempora & frontem
affuerit. At fanguinis eruptio magis expectanda venit in his, qui nundum quintum & trigefimum annum attigerunt.
In fenioribus verò fuppuratio. *Prænot.*
129.

§ LVI. Caput dolenti, & vehementer laboranti, pus aut aqua, aut fanguis
per nares, os, aut aures effluens, morbum folvit. *Aph.* VI. 10.

Ex Delirio.

§ LVII. In quovis morbó valere ratione, & rectè fe ad ea quæ offeruntur
habere,

habere, bonum. Contrarium verò, malum. *Aph.* II. 33.

§ LVIII. In acutis rectus oculorum intuitus ac motûs pernicitas, fomnus turbulentus, pervigilium, interdumque fanguinis è naribus ftillatio, nihil boni denunciant, *Coac.* 227.

§ LIX. In febribus ardentibus aurium tinnitus, visûs hebetudo, narium gravitas, in delirium præcipitant, nifi fanguis è naribus proruperit. *Ibid.* 131.

§ LX. Facere aliquid præter confuetudinem, velut inftituere, velleque ea quæ priùs non confueverat, aut contrarium iis quæ fuerant confueta, malum & dementiæ proximum. *Coac.* 47.

§ LXI. Screatio frequens. fi quod aliud fignum accefferit phrenitidis nuncia. *Ibid.* 244.

§ LXII. In cephalagiâ, vomitus æruginofi, cum furditate, & fomni vacuitate,

tate, infaniam brevi denunciant. *Ibid.*
169.

§ LXIII. Quibus pellucidæ & albæ
funt urinæ, malum. Maximè verò
tales in phreneticis apparent. *Aph.*
IV. 72.

§ LXIV. In ventrem jacere ei qui per
bonam valetudinem ita dormire minimè
confuevit, delirium, aut partium circa
ventrem dolorem arguit. *Præn.* 13.

§ LXV. Ab homine moderato ferox re-
fponfio, & vox acuta, malum portendunt.
Coac. 51.

§ LXVI. Flatum abfque fono & ftrepitu trajici per inferiora, optimum. Meliùs autem fuerit ipfum cum fono tranfire
quàm furfum revolvi: quamvis ita tra-
jectus denunciet indè vexari hominem,
aut delirare; nifi prudens ac fciens talem
flatûs exitum moliatur. *Præn.* 68.

§ LXVII.

§ LXVII. Deliria quæ cum risu fiunt,
tutiora. Quæ vero studio adhibito, peri-
culosiora. *Aph.* VI. 53.

§ LXVIII. Quicumque supra quadraginta annos phrenetici fiunt, non ita
valdè sani evadunt. Minus enim periclitantur quorum naturæ & ætati morbus
magis affinis fuerit. *Ibid.* VIII. 91.

§ LXIX. Ubi delirium somnus sedave-
rit, bonum. *Aph.* II. 2.

§ LXX. Phrænetici parum bibunt,
ex levi strepitu facilè irritantur, tremuli
sunt, & facilè convelluntur. *Coac.* 96.

§ LXXI. Contremiscere simul ac
stultè palpare manibus, phreneticum.
Coac. 76.

§ LXXII. De manuum motione ita
censeo: in febribus acutis, aut pulmo-
num inflammationibus, aut phrenitide,
aut capitis doloribus, quibus ante faciem
feruntur, & aliquid frustrà venantur, &
festu-

féstucas colligunt, aut floccos à vestibus
evellunt, & ex pariete paleas carpunt;
ex his omnibus malum & mortem por-
tendi. *Præn.* 17.

§ LXXIII. Qui cum silentio, nec tamen
aphoni, à potestate mentis exeunt; lethale.
Coac. 65.

§ LXXIV. Quæ circa res necessarias
versantur deliria, pessima: indèque si ingravescant mortifera. *Coac.* 98.

§ LXXV. Qui ad manum exiliunt,
malo sunt loco. *Coac.* 59.

§ LXXVI. Cervicis dolor cum in
omni febre terrificus, tum verò morti-
ferus iis qui sunt in metu insaniæ.
Ibid. 273.

§ LXXVII. Quibus jam desperatis le-
vis tremor incidit & æruginosa vomitio,
mors propè est. *Ibid.* 62.

F f § LXXVIII.

§ LXXVIII. Egregie phreniticorum tremores citam mortem denunciant. *Ibid.* 97.

§ LXXIX. Dentium collisio aut stridor præter consuetudinem à teneris contractam, insaniam, ac mortem denunciant. Quod si jam deliranti id accidat, prorsus lethale. Quin & dentes resiccari perniciem denotat. *Ibid.* 235.

§ LXXX. Deliria cum fixâ virium exolutione, funesta. *Ibid.* 100.

§ LXXXI. Crebræ in phreneticis cum perfrictione sputationes nigrorum vomitionem prænunciant. *Ibid.* 102.

Oblivio insensibilitas.

§ LXXXII. A rigore familiares non agnoscere, malum. Oblivio item mala. *Coac.* 6.

§ LXXXIII.

§ LXXXIII. Qui aliquâ corporis parte dolentes, ferè dolorem non sentiunt ; iis mens ægrotat. *Aph.* II. 6.

§ LXXXIV. Omnino malum denunciat quæ in acutâ febre immeritò sitis extincta est. *Coac.* 58.

§ LXXXV. Exitiosa alvi dejectio quæ sensum ægri fallit. *Coac.* 631.

§ LXXXVI. Perniciosa est urina quæ inscio ægro redditur. *Coac.* 580.

§ LXXXVII. Quibuscumque in ægritudinibus oculi ex voluntate lacrymantur, bonum. Quibus verò citra voluntatem, malum. *Aph.* IV. 52. VII. 81.

Somnus vigilia.

§ LXXXVIII. Noctu dormiendum, vigilandum interdiù. *Præn.* 53. Pessimum verò si neque noctu dormiat, neque interdiù. Nam aut ob dolorem vigilia

adest,

adest, aut delirii affuturi hæc est nota.
Ibid. 56.

§ LXXXIX. Quo in morbo somnus
noxam affert lethale. Si verò somnus
prosit, minimè lethale. *Aph.* II. 1.

§ XC. In vigiliâ convulsio aut delirium,
malum. *Aph.* II. 3. VII. 18.

Ex soporosis affectibus.

§ XCI. An sopor ubique malum.
Coac. 178.

§ XCII. Apoplexia repente oborta
solubilis, febri diuturnæ superveniens
mortifera. *Ibid.* 480.

§ XCIII. Si quis in febre fandi sit impotens: malo est loco. *Ibid.* 34.

§ XCIV. Quæ cum exolutione soporosâ
fiunt aphoniæ: lethales. *Ibid.* 250.

§ XCV.

§ XCV. Vocis defectio unà cum virium exolutione, peſſima. *Ibid.* 245.

§ XCVI. Somni veternoſi, unàque al-
ſioſi, mortiferi. *Coac.* 181.

§ XCVII. Parotides ſymptomaticæ
pravæ paraplecticis. *Ibid.* 202.

§ XCVIII. Qui ex dolore fiunt aphoni,
crudeliter moriuntur. *Ibid.* 249.

§ XCIX. Qui dormiendo efflant, ac
projectos artus aut etiam retractos oſten-
dunt, conniventque oculis; malo ſunt
loco. *Coac.* 64.

§ C. Qui ex lethargo evadunt, magnâ
ex parte ſuppurantur. *Ibid.* 140.

Ex affectionibus convulſivis.

§ CI. Quæ cadunt in hyſtericas ſine
febre convulſiones, faciles. *Coac.* 349.

§ CII.

adeſt, aut delirii affuturi hæc eſt nota. *Ibid.* 56.

§ LXXXIX. Quo in morbo ſomnus noxam affert lethale. Si verò ſomnus profit, minimè lethale. *Aph.* II. 1.

§ XC. In vigiliâ convulſio aut delirium, malum. *Aph.* II. 3. VII. 18.

Ex ſoporofis affeEtibus.

§ XCI. An ſopor ubique malum. *Coac.* 178.

§ XCII. Apoplexia repente oborta ſolubilis, febri diuturnæ ſuperveniens mortifera. *Ibid.* 480.

§ XCIII. Si quis in febre fandi ſit impotens: malo eſt loco. *Ibid.* 34.

§ XCIV. Quæ cum exolutione ſoporosâ ſiunt aphoniæ: lethales. *Ibid.* 250.

§ XCV.

§ XCV. Vocis defectio unà cum virium exolutione, peffima. *Ibid.* 245.

§ XCVI. Somni veternofi, unàque alfiofi, mortiferi. *Coac.* 181.

§ XCVII. Parotides fymptomaticæ pravæ paraplecticis. *Ibid.* 202.

§ XCVIII. Qui ex dolore fiunt aphoni, crudeliter moriuntur. *Ibid.* 249.

§ XCIX. Qui dormiendo efflant, ac projectos artus aut etiam retractos oftendunt, conniventque oculis; malo funt loco. *Coac.* 64.

§ C. Qui ex lethargo evadunt, magnâ ex parte fuppurantur. *Ibid.* 140.

Ex affectionibus convulfivis.

§ CI. Quæ cadunt in hyftericas fine febre convulfiones, faciles. *Coac.* 349.

§ CII.

§ CII. Quibus oculi fcintillant valde intenti, nec funt apud fe, & convelluntur. *Ibid.* 351.

§ CIII. Puerulis convulfiones incidunt, fi febris acuta fuerit, alvus claufa, fomni fint expertes, & terreantur & ejularint, tum etiam fi colorem mutent, ac pallido, vel livido, aut etiam rubro fuffundantur. Hæ (convulfiones) facilè incidunt puerulis nuper natis, ad feptimum ætatis annum. At grandiores pueri, & viri non adeò per febres convulfionibus prehenduntur, nifi vehementiffimum ac peffimum aliquod fignum ex his quæ in phrenetide fieri folent affuerit. *Præn.* 151, 152. Eadem ferè. *Coac.* 109.

§ CIV. Febrem convulfioni fupervenire fatiùs eft, quam febri convulfionem. *Aph.* II. 26.

§ CV. Spasmo aut tetano vexato febris fi accefferit, morbum folvit. *Aph.* IV. 57.

§ CVI.

§ CVI. Convulsionem & nervorum diſtentionem ſuperveniens febris ſolvit. *Coac.* 354.

§ CVII. Convulsio febri ſuperveniens funeſta : minimum verò puerulis. *Ibid.* 356.

§ CVIII. Qui ſeptem annis provectiores ſunt, convulſione non tentantur in febre. Sin autem deſperati. *Ibid.* 357.

§ CIX. Si febre detento collum repentè obverſum fuerit, & vix deglutire potuerit, tumore non exiſtente in faucibus ; lethale. *Aph.* IV. 35.

§ CX. Convulsiones cum febre acutâ, funeſtæ. *Coac.* 269.

§ CXI. Cum opiſtothono rigor necat. *Coac.* 23.

§ CXII. Fauces valdè dolentes & æquales cum jactatione, crudeliter & citò mortiferæ. *Coac.* 265.

§ CXIII.

§ CXIII. Faucium dolor prægrandis parotides & convulsiones facit, atque cervicis & dorsi dolores. *Coac.* 268.

§ CXIV. Cervicis duritas & dolor prægrandis, maxillarum item connexio, venarum jugularium pulsus fortis, unàque tendinum contentio; hæc sunt mortifera. *Ibid.* 261.

§ CXV. Dentium collisio aut stridor præter consuetudinem. *Vid. supra* 79.

§ CXVI. Convulsio ab elleboro lethalis. *Aph.* V. 1.

§ CXVII. Convulsio vulneri superveniens, lethalis. *Ibid.* 2.

§ CXVIII. A copioso sanguinis fluxu singultus aut convulsio, malum. *Ibid.* 3.

§ CXIX. A purgatione immodicâ convulsio aut singultus, malum. *Ibid.* 4.

§ CXX.

§ CXX. In fluxu muliebri convulſio & animi deliquium ſi accedat, malum. *Ibid.* 56.

§ CXXI. A vomitu ſingultus & oculi rubicundi, malum. *Aph.* VII. 3.

§ CXXII. Inflammationi hepatis, ſingultus ſi ſupervenerit, malum. *Ibid.* 17.

§ CXXIII. Qui tetano corripiuntur intra quatuor dies intereunt, ſi verò hos effugerint ſani evadunt. *Aph.* V. 6.

Ex Surditate.

§ CXXIV. In acutis obſurdeſcere, furioſum. *Coac.* 196.

§ CXXV. In acutis & turbulentis morbis obveniens ſurditas, malum. *Ibid.* 190.

§ CXXVI. Gravi ſurditate tentati, dum aliquid prehendunt tremuli, linguæ

G g   reſorefolutione, ac torpore affecti, malè habere judicantur. *Coac.* 197.

Solutiones morborum acutorum fpontaneæ.

§ CXXVII. At verò morbi acuti, judicantur fanguine è naribus tempeftivâ crifi prorumpente, fudore item multo, atque purulentâ urinâ & vitreâ laudabili preditâ hypoftafi, quæ cumulatìm funditur, tum abfceffu etiam memorabili, nec non mucosâ & cruentâ alvo repentè citatâ, poftremò vomitionibus minimè malis in crifi. *Coac.* 150.

Ex Vomitu.

§ CXXVIII. Si quis in febre non lethali dixerit fibi caput dolere, aut oculorum aciem caligine quâdam perftringi, & ftomachi dolor accefferit, tum vomitio aderit. Si verò etiam rigor accefferit, &

inferiores

inferiores hypochondrii partes frigidas ha-
buerit, adhùc citiùs evomet. *Præn.* 144.

§ CXXIX. Qui vomituri funt, priùs
illi falivant. *Coac.* 566.

§ CXXX. Si cui (febricitanti) inquie-
tudines, cordis morfus, & crebra fputatio:
in procinctu vomitio eft. *Ibid.* 142.

§ CXXXI. Vomitus per quam utilis
eft qui pituitâ & bile permixtus eft, nec
admodum craffus, nec multus. Nam
meraciores pejores funt. Sin autem id
quod vomitione excluditur, aut porra-
ceum fit, aut lividum, aut nigrum;
quamcumque horum colorum fpeciem
referat, in pravis habere oportet. Quod
fi omnes illos colores idem homo vomitione exhibeat: valdè quidem id lethale eft. Sed mortem in propinquo effe
fignificat lividus ille vomitus qui tetrum
odorem fpirat. Nam omnes fub putridi
& graveolentes odores in iis omnibus quæ
vomitu rejiciuntur, mali funt. *Præn.* 81,
2, 83, 84, 85.

G g 2 § CXXXII.

§ CXXXII. Morbis quibus vis incipientibus, si atrabilis suprà infràve exierit lethale. *Aph.* IV. 22.

§ CXXXIII. Bilis vomitus vulneri succedens, malum denunciat, præcipuèque in capitis vulneribus. *Coac.* 507.

§ CXXXIV. Qui cum anxietate citra vomitum exacerbantur, malum. Tum quos lacessit nausea sine vomitu. *Coac.* 557.

§ CXXXV. Vomitiones exiguæ, biliosæ, malum : tum præcipuè si pervigilio conflictentur ægri. *Ibid.* 558.

§ CXXXVI. In meris vomitionibus lethalis singultus, item convulsio. Similiter & in purgationum excessu quem inferunt medicamenta. *Ibid.* 565.

Ex alvi dejectione.

§ CXXXVII. Alvi dejectio optima, si mollis est & consistat, eoque tempore quo per sanitatem dejici solet : copiâ verò ciborum

borum ingeſtorum rationi reſponderit.
Talis enim exitus inferiorem alvum benè
valere declarat. *Præn.* 57.

§ CXXXVIII. Quod ſi liquida fuerit
conſentaneum eſt ipſam neque ſtridere,
neque paucum & crebro excerni. Frequens enim deſidendi labor ægrum fati-
gat, eique vigilias adfert. *Ibid.* 58.

§ CXXXIX. Quod ſi affatim & ſæpè
dejicit, periculum eſt ne in animi deliquium incidat. *Ibid.* 59.

§ CXL. Crassiorem fieri dejectionem
oportet, morbo ad criſim properante.
Ibid. 61.

§ CXLI. Sit etiam ſubruſa, nec admodùm graveolens. *Ibid.*

§ CXLII. Expedit etiam lumbricos
teretes unà cum excrementis alvi de-
ſcendere, morbo ad criſim properante.
Ibid. 62.

§ CXLIII.

§ CXLIII. Valdè aquofa, aut alba, aut pallida, aut prærubra, aut fpumans, calamitofa. *Ibid.* 64.

§ CXLIV. Mala etiam quæ exigua, glutinofa, fubflava & æqualis exiftit. *Ibid.* 65.

§ CXLV. His verò magis funefta quæ nigra, aut pinguis, aut livida, aut æru-ginofa, aut graveolens. *Ibid.* 66.

§ CXLVI. Qui nigra egerunt, frigidum illi exudant. *Coac.* 618.

§ CXLVII. Dejectiones variæ majorem quam illæ diuturnitatis fpem afferunt, fed tamen non minus funt funeftæ : hujufmodi funt ftrigmentofæ, biliofæ, cruentæ, porraceæ, & nigræ, five fecedant fimul, five aliæ poft alias. *Præn.* 67.

§ CXLVIII. In febre ardente fi alvus profufe feratur, mortiferum. *Coac.* 129.

§ CXLIX.

§ CXLIX. LIQUIDA frequenſque deje&io, ſive multa, ſive pauca, malum; hæc enim vigilias, illa etiam virium exolutionem parit. *Coac.* 609.

§ CL. DYSENTERIA, ſi ab atrabile inceperit, lethalis. *Aph.* IV. 24.

§ CLI. Sɪ à dyſenteriâ occupato veluti carnes ſubierint, lethale. *Ibid.* 26.

§ CLII. SANGUINEM ſuperne quidem ferri qualiſcumque ſit, malum: inferne verò niger ſi dejiciatur, bonum. *Ibid.* 25.

§ CLIII. SANGUIS ſincerus alvo per feceſſum reje&us, malo eſt: præſertìm ſi dolor aliquis adſit. *Coac.* 605.

§ CLIV. A SUPPRESSIONE alvi, meteoriſmus hypochondriorum gravis: maximè verò iis qui ab inveteratione tabeſcunt, & quibus alvi profusè ferebantur. *Coac.* 301.

§ CLV.

§ CLV. In iis qui longo tempore con-
sumpti sunt, temeraria alvi exolutio unà
cum vocis defectione & tremore, lethalis.
Ibid. 634.

Ex Urinis.

§ CLVI. Urina optima est, ubi & alba
hypostasis & lævis & æqualis per omne
tempus, quoad morbus judicatus fuerit.
Talis enim ad securitatem & brevitatem
morbi præclare apparet. *Præn.* 70.

§ CLVII. Urina in febre quæ albam
& lævem habet hypostasim, atque con-
stantem, citam illius dimissionem ostendit.
Coac. 575.

§ CLVIII. Quibus urina cito hypostasim habet, celeriter illi judicantur.
Ibid. 598.

§ CLIX. Sin talis sit urinæ intermissio
quædam, ut modò pura reddatur, modo
hypostasis alba & lævis subsidat; diutur-
nior

nior quidem eſt morbus, & minus res
ægri in tuto ſunt. *Præn.* 71.

§ CLX. Sɪɴ ſubrubra reddatur urina
cum hypoſtaſi lævi & æquali, diuturnioris
quidem morbi ea erit quam illa jam me-
morata, ſed admodum ſalutaris. *Ibid.* 72.

§ CLXI. Qᴜᴇ in urinis farinæ craſſioris
ſpeciem hypoſtaſes referunt, pravæ; his
multo pejores ſunt lamineæ; albæ verò
& tenues admodùm ſunt perniciofæ; ſed
his omnibus magis funeſtæ ſunt furfura-
ceæ. *Ibid.* 73.

§ CLXII. Aᴛ verò nebulæ in urinis,
albæ quidem & verſus fundum utiles.
Rubræ autem & nigræ, item lividæ, dif-
ficiles. *Coac.* 577.

§ CLXIII. Qᴜᴀɴᴅɪᴜ autem fuerit urina rubra & tenuis, morbum adhuc pepaſ-
mi expertem ſignificat. Quod ſi diu talis reddatur, periculum eſt ne vires ægri
valere non poſſint donec urina mitificata
fuerit. *Præn.* 75.

H h   CLXIV.

§ CLXIV. Inter urinas funeſtiſſimæ
ſunt graveolentes, aqueæ, nigræ, & craſſæ.
Ibid. 76.

§ CLXV. Sed tum viris, tum mulieri-
bus nigræ peſſimæ; pueris verò aqueæ.
Ibid. 77.

§ CLXVI. Pestifera eſt ea quæ & hy-
poſta.ſm habet nigram, & ipſa quoque nigra eſt. *Coac.* 580.

§ CLXVII. Aquosa verò & alba, in
diuturnis morbis perſeverans, difficil-
lem & non ſecuram judicationem facit.
Coac. 576.

§ CLXVIII. Urinæ derepente præter
rationem parum concoctæ, vitioſæ ſunt.
Atque omnino quidquid præter rationem
coctum eſt in acuto, malum. *Coac.* 579.

§ CLXIX. Peripneumonicis pernicio-
ſa eſt quæ initio coctionem exibet, verum poſt quartum diem tenuis evadit.
Coac. 580.

§ CLXX.

§ CLXX. PLEURITICIS urina cruenta, obfcura cum variâ hypoftafi & indifcretâ, ut plurimum intra dies quatuordecim mortem affert. Sed illud confeftim mortiferum eft in pleuriticis, urinam reddi porraceam cum nigrâ hypoftafi aut furfuraceâ. *Coac.* 581.

Ex Sudore.

§ CLXXI. SUDORES optimi quidem per omnes morbos acutos, qui diebus judicatoriis contingunt, & penitùs febre liberant. *Præn.* 22.

§ CLXXII. BONI verò quicumque toto corpore oriuntur, faciuntque ut æger morbum faciliùs ferre videatur. *Ibid.* 23.

§ CLXXIII. AT qui nihil tale efficiunt, minimè funt utiles. *Ibid.*

§ CLXXIV. PESSIMI autem frigidi, quique circa caput tantummodò, faciem & cervicem exoriuntur. Ii namque cum

acutâ

acutâ febre mortem, cum mitiore verò mórbi longitudinem prænuntiant. *Ibid.*24.

§ CLXXV. Similiter & qui in toto corpore eodem quo & in capite modo proveniunt. *Ibid.* 25.

§ CLXXVI. Qui verò milii formam referunt, & circa cervicem, tantùm oboriuntur, pravi. *Ibid.* 26.

§ CLXXVII. Sudores boni funt qui guttatim, & cum exhalatione fiunt. *Ibid.* 27.

§ CLXXVIII. Causus rigore accedente folvitur. *Coac.* 135.

§ CLXXIX. In acutis exudantes tenuiter & anxii, malum. *Coac.* 53.

Ex narium hemorrhagiâ.

§ CLXXX. At verò quibus in febre continuâ caput dolet, & fuffufionis caliginofæ

ginofæ loco hebefcunt oculi, aut etiam
ignes micant ex oculis, & cardialagiæ loco, dextrà aut finiftrâ hypochondriorum
parte diftentio quædam percipitur, doloris & inflammationis expers, his narium
profluvium vomitionis loco jamjam adfu-
turum fpes eft. Sed juvenibus potiùs
illud expeclandum eft. Iis verò qui
trigefimum annum attigerint, & fenioribus, minùs. *Præn.* 149.

§ CLXXXI. Si cui febricitanti rubor
in facie luceat, unàque capitis dolor prægrandis, & venarum emicet pulfus; ferè
profluvium fanguinis è naribus indè venit. *Coac.* 142.

§ CLXXXII. Qui dolore capitis gravi
ad finciput affliguntur, fomni expertes,
fanguinem profundunt è naribus, præ-
fertim fi quid in cervice contendatur.
Coac. 168.

§ CLXXXIII. Per exigua ftillicidia,
malum. *Coac.* 57.

§ CLXXXIV.

§ CLXXXIV. A sanguinis fluxu, delirium, aut etiam convulsio, malum.
Aph. VII. 9.

§ CLXXXV. Morbus regius si antè
diem septimum accèsserit, malum signi-
ficat; septimo autem, nono, undecimo,
ac decimo quarto, judicationem affert.
Dum hypochondrium non induret. Si
secus contingat, res in dubium vertitur.
Coac. 121.

Ex Parotidibus.

§ CLXXXVI. Inter acutos parotides
potissimum in causis assurgunt, ac tum si
febrem lege criticâ non expellant, nec
ipsæ coquantur, nec sanguis fundatur è
naribus, nec verò urinæ excipiant cras-
sam hypostasim, moriuntur. Sed ab-
scessus ejusmodi non raro antè residunt.
Coac. 207.

§ CLXXXVII. Sed & tum febres
considerare oportet num ingravescant,
an

an vero mitefcant: atque ita pronunciare. *Ibid.*

§ CLXXXVIII. Quæ dolenter ad aurem affurgunt, peftifera. *Coac.* 199.

§ CLXXXIX. Sī cui ex febre ardente venit parotis quæ purulenta non fiat, haud facilè fuperftes evadit. *Coac.* 138.

§ CXC. Ex glandularum tumoribus febres omnes malæ funt, exceptis diariis. *Aph.* IV. 55.

§ CXCI. Quī per febres laffitudinem fentiunt, iis ad articulos & juxta maxillas potiffimùm abfceffus fiunt. *Aph.* IV. 31.

§ CXCII. Quibus fub judicationis tempus juxta aures exorta tubercula minimè fuppurant, iis fubfidentibus, morbi reverfionem fieri contingit. *Lib. de hum.* 77.

Abfcefsûs

Abfcefsûs prævifio.

§ CXCIII. Quos febres longæ exercent, iis vel tubercula ad articulos, vel dolores fiunt. *Aph.* IV. 44.

§ CXCIV. In longâ febre, falutariter tamen affecto ægro; fi neque ob inflammationem aliquam, nec ob ullam aliam evidentem occafionem dolor detinet; in hoc abfceffus cum tumore, aut dolore ad articulum aliquem expectandus, maximéque in inferioribus locis. Hujufmodi abfceffus magis contingere folent & breviori tempore iis qui trigefimum annum nondum attigerunt. Minimè fenioribus. *Præn.* 139.

§ CXCV. Attendendum verò ftatim ad abfcefsûs figna, fi viginti dies febris detinens fuperat. Hujufmodi autem abfceffus expectandus, ubi febris continua eft. *Ibid.* 140.

§ CXCVI,

§ CXCVI. In quartanam verò firmari debere, ubi intermiferit, & errabundum in modum prehenderit, & ita ad autumnum deducatur. *Ibid.* 141.

§ CXCVII. Quibus fpes eft abfceffum fore ad articulos, eos abfceffu liberat urina multa, & craffa, & alba. . . . Si verò etiam fanguis è naribus proruperit, brevi admodùm folvit. *Aph.* IV. 74.

§ CXCVIII. Febricitantium non omninò leviter, permanere, & nihil minui corpus, aut etiam magis quàm pro ratione colliquari, malum. Illud enim morbi longitudinem, hoc verò debilitatem fignificat. *Aph.* II. 28.

Ex Metaftafi.

§ CXCIX. Erisipelas in anginâ intùs foras converti utile, at foris intùs, mortiferum. Intùs verò convertitur, cum rubore evanefcente pectus gravatur, ac difficiliùs fpirat æger. *Coac.* 366.

I i

CC.

§ CC. Lumborum & inferiorum partium dolores qui cum febre affligunt, fi iis relictis, feptum tranfverfum invadant, exitiales admodùm funt. Adhibere igitur animum oportet cæteris fignis, ut fi quod aliorum fignorum pravum appareat, omni fpe deftituatur homo. *Præn.* 118.

§ CCI. Si verò irruente ad feptum tranfverfum morbo, non alia prava figna fuperveniant: fuppuratum hunc fore multa fpes fit. *Ibid.* 120.

§ CCII. Anginâ detento tumorem fieri in collo bonum. Foras enim morbus vertitur. *Aph.* VI. 37.

§ CCIII. Quibus in febris affiduitate puftulæ toto corpore fuboriuntur, mortiferum illud eft, nifi purulento abfceffu, qui hic potiffimùm ad aures erumpit, periculo defungantur. *Coac.* 114.

Ex

Ex Livedine & Gangræná.

§ CCIV. Livedines in febre mortem proximam denunciant. *Coac.* 66.

§ CCV. Præter gravitatem (corporis) fi ungues & digiti livefcant, mors confeftìm expectanda eft. *Præn.* 50.

§ CCVI. At omnino nigri, tum digiti, tum pedes, minùs quàm liventes, periculofi funt. Sed alia etiam figna confideranda. Si enim facilè malum ferre videatur, & aliud quoddam ex falubribus fignis adfuerit, morbus ad abfceffum vergit: ita ut æger morbo quidem fupereffe, & partes corporis dénigratæ decidere debeant. *Ibid.* 51.

Ex Cute.

§ CCVII. Caput manus & pedes frigere, ventre & lateribus calentibus, malum denunciat. *Præn.* 46.

§ CCVIII.

§ CCVIII At corpus totum æqualiter calidum effe ac molle, optimum. *Ibid.* 47.

§ CCIX. In acutis frigiditas extremarum partium, malum. *Aph.* VII. 1.

§ CCX. Ex dolore forti partium circa ventrem, frigiditas extremarum partium, malum. *Aph.* VII. 26.

§ CCXI. In acutâ febre exteriora perfrigerari, interiora verò fic uri ut fitìm faciant, malum. *Coac.* 115.

Coctionis figna.

§ CCXII. Concoctiones celeritatem judicationis, & fanitatis fecuritatem oftendunt. *Epid.* 1.

§ CCXIII. Crassiorem fieri dejectionem oportet, morbo ad judicationem properante. *Præn.* 61.

§ CCXIV.

§ CCXIV. Quibus feptimâ die crifis contingit, iis urina rubram die quartâ nubeculam habet, aliaque pro ratione. *Aph.* IV. 71.

§ CCXV. Quibus in urinis citò aliquid fubfidet, hi brevi judicantur. *Coac.* 598.

§ CCXVI. Oculorum claritas ac eorum album ex nigro aut livido clarum fieri, ad judicationem confert. Ac quo celeriùs clarefcunt, eo celeriorem judicationem, at tardiùs, tardiorem fignificant. *Coac.* 217.

§ CCXVII. Judicatoria non judicantia, partìm lethalia funt, partìm difficilis judicationis. *Epid. lib.* 2. *fec.* 1.

§ CCXVIII. Quæ in febribus fruftra abfcefsûs fpem fac unt, maligna. *Coac.* 145.

§ CCXIX. Iis quæ fine ratione levantur, non fidendum. Nec formidanda mala quæ præter rationem contingunt. Pluri-

ma

ma enim horum incerta funt; nec admodum perſeverare, aut longo tempore du-
rare conſueverunt. *Aph.* II. 27.

§ CCXX. Q U Æ cum pravis ſignis mi-
teſcunt, & quæ cum bonis non remittunt,
moleſta ſunt & difficilia. *Coac.* 48.

Quibus præcipuè ſignis morbi acuti
ſalutares, aut periculoſi dignoſcan-
tur.

§ CCXXI. Q U I ex morbo evaſuri ſunt,
facilè ſpirant, dolore vacant, noctu dor-
miunt, aliaque ſecuriſſima habent ſigna.
Præn. 126.

§ CCXXII. A T perituri difficultate ſpirandi vexantur, delirant, vigilant, cæte-
raque peſſima habent ſigna. *Ibid.* 127.

§ CCXXIII. Q U Æ ex dorſi dolore principia morborum ducuntur, difficilia.
Coac. 309.

§ CCXXIV.

§ CCXXIV. Delassatis in febribus, ad articulos, & circa maxillas maximè abfceſſus fiunt. *Aph.* IV. 31.

§ CCXXV. Convulsio in febre, manuum & pedum dolores maligni, maligna etiam doloris à femore furfum irruptio; nec à genuum dolore levatio ulla fperabilis. Quin & furarum dolores & mentis emotiones maligni. *Coac.* 30.

§ CCXXVI. Delassati, caliginoſi, vigiles, comatoſi, æftu incandefcentes, malè habent. *Coac.* 35.

Convalefcentia firma, aut inſtabilis.

§ CCXXVII. Somni arctiores placidi, firmam criſim denunciant : tumultuoſi, laborioſi, inſtabilem. *Coac.* 151.

§ CCXXVIII. A morbo belle comedenti, nihil proficere corpus, malum. *Aph.* II. 31.

§ CCXXIX.

§ CCXXIX. Quibus febres ceſſant, neque apparentibus ſolutionis ſignis, nec diebus judicatoriis; iis recidiva expectanda eſt. *Præn.* 138.

§ CCXXX. Qui diuturno defuncti morbo ex animi ſententiâ cibum capiunt, nec proficiunt, graviſſimè relabuntur. *Coac.* 127.

§ CCXXXI. Morborum reverſionibus tentantur, quibus febre ſolutis vehementes vigiliæ, aut turbulenti ſomni, aut corporis robur ſolvitur, aut ſingulorum membrorum adſunt dolores; & quibus febres non accedentibus ſolutionis ſignis, neque diebus judicatoriis quieſcunt. *Lib. de criſib.*

§ CCXXXII. Stomachi dolor & pulſus hypochondriorum, febre extinctâ, malum denunciant: idque cum aliàs, tum in ſudatiunculâ. *Coac.* 283.

§ CCXXXIII.

§ CCXXXIII. Quæ longo tempore extenuantur corpora, lente reficere oportet; quæ verò-brevi, celeriter. *Aph.* II. 7.

Circa morbos prægnantium & puerperarum.

§ CCXXXIV. Mulierem gravidam morbo quopiam acuto corripi, lethale. *Aph.* V. 30.

§ CCXXXV. Mulieri utero gerenti, si àlvus multùm fluxerit, periculum est ne abortiat. *Ibid.* 34.

§ CCXXXVI. Si prægnanti tenesmus supervenerit, abortum facit. *Aph.* VII. 27.

§ CCXXXVII. Quæcumque utero habentes febribus corripiuntur, & fortiter attenuantur sine manifestâ occasione, difficulter pariunt & periculosè, aut abortum facientes, periclitantur. *Aph.* V. 55.

K k   § CCXXXVIII.

§ CCXXXVIII. Ante partum sub indè rigere, & citra dolorem parturire, periculosum. *Coac.* 538.

§ CCXXXIX. Uterinæ duritates in alvo admodùm dolorificæ, crudeliter atque citò perniciosæ. *Coac.* 528.

§ CCXL. Quæ ex partu & abortu copiosa, celeriter, cum impetu feruntur, si subsistant, molestiam exhibent. His rigor inimicus, & alvi perturbatio, præcipuè verò si doleant hypochondrium. *Coac.* 516.

Crises.

§ CCXLI. Quibus crisis sit, his nox accessionem præcedens gravis, subsequens verò levior plerumque. *Aph.* II. 13.

Dies

Dies decretorii.

§ CCXLII. Febricitantem nifi die-bus imparibus febris reliquerit, folet re-verti. *Aph.* IV. 61.

§ CCXLIII. Quibus in febribus quo-tidie rigores fiunt, quotidie folvuntur. *Ibid.* 63. Quæ paribus diebus exacer-bantur, paribus judicantur. Quorum au-tem exacerbationes in imparibus fiunt, ea in imparibus judicantur. Eft autem pri-mus judicatorius, ex circuitibus diebus paribus judicantibus, quartus dies, deinde fextus, decimus, decimus-quartus, deci-mus-octavus, vigefimus; fed ex circuiti-bus verò in imparibus diebus judicanti-bus, primus eft dies tertius, deinde quin-tus, feptimus, nonus, undecimus, deci-mus-feptimus, vigefimus-primus, vigefi-mus-feptimus, trigefimus-primus. *Epid. lib.* 1. *fect.* 3.

§ CCXLIV. Sudores febricitantibus boni funt & judicatoris qui cæperint die

3, 5, 7, 9, 11, 14, 17, 21, 27, 31, 34.
Aph. IV. 36.

§ CCXLV. Febres judicantur die 4,
7, 11, 14, 17, 21. *De dieb. decret.*

§ CCXLVI. Septimi quartus index.
Alterius feptimanæ, octavus eft initium.
Notandus verò undecimus: is enim quartus eft alterius feptimanæ. Notandus
rursùm decimus-feptimus. Hic enim eft
quartus quidem à decimo-quarto, feptimus verò ab undecimo. *Aph.* II. 24.

§ CCXLVII. Febrium judicationes iifdem numerantur diebus, quibus & evadunt, & moriuntur homines. Nam &
mitiffimæ, & quæ fecuriffimis incedunt
fignis, die quarto, aut antè definunt.
Maximè verò malignæ, & quæ cum gra-
viffimis fignis fiunt, quarto vel priùs inter-
ficiunt. Primus itaque earum infultus ad
hunc modum definit, fecundus ad feptimum, tertius ad undecimum, quartus
ad decimum-quartum, quintus ad deci-
mum-

mum-feptimum, fextus ad vigefimum.
Præn. 122.

§ CCXLVIII. N e q u e verò horum
quicquam integris diebus numerari po-
teft. *Ibid.* 123.

De Pleuritide & Peripneumoniâ.

§ CCXLIX. E x e r c i t a t a & denfa
corpora celeriùs à plueritide & peripneumoniâ intereunt quam otio dedita. *Coac.*
398.

§ CCL. P l e u r i t i c i s dolores & alvum
emolliri utile; fputa colorari, nullos in
pectore ftrepitus fieri, urinam rectè procedere. Eorum contraria difficilia funt,
& fputum dulcefcere. *Coac.* 386.

§ CCLI. L a t e r i s dolor, in fputo biliofo, qui immeritò vanuit, infaniam facit.
Ibid. 418.

§ CCLII.

§ CCLII. Duobus doloribus fimul fi-
entibus, non fecundùm eundem locum,
vehementior obfcurat alterum. *Aph.*
II. 46.

§ CCLIII. Quibus autem pleuriticis
initio quidem dolores funt mites, quintâ
aut fextâ die ingravefcunt, ferè ad duo-
decimum perveniunt, raroque fervantur.
Coac. 387.

§ CCLIV. Terrificæ funt pleuritides,
in quibus dolorifica fursùm funt mala.
Coac. 381.

§ CCLV. Spirationes quæ non nifi
erectâ cervice ducuntur, dirum hydropem
faciunt. *Ibid.* 424.

§ CCLVI. Siccæ pleuritides, & fputi
expertes graviffimæ. *Coac.* 381.

§ CCLVII. At verò fputum in pleuriticis fi tertiâ die maturari, & expui cœperit, citas facit folutiones: fi feriùs tar-
diores. *Ibid.* 385.

§ CCLVIII.

§ CCLVIII. Expectoratum verò in omnibus morbis qui in pulmones & latera incidunt, citò & expeditè expectorari de_bet, sputoque flavum valdè permixtum apparere. *Prog.* 86.

§ CCLIX. Etenim si multò post morbi principium expectoretur, aut flavum quid aut rufum, aut quod multam tussim affe-rat, nec exquisite permixtum sit: deterius est. *Ibid.* 87.

§ CCLX. Flavum quippe si since_rum fuerit, periculum subesse testatur. *Ibid.* 84.

§ CCLXI. Album autem, & viscidum, & rotundum, inutile. *Ibid.* 89.

§ CCLXII. Malum quoque valdè vi-ride, aut pallidum, aut spumans. *Ibid.* 90.

§ CCLXIII. At si adeò sincerum fuerit ut etiam nigrum appareat, id illis deteri-us est. *Ibid.* 91.

§ CCLXIV.

§ CCLXIV. Malum quoque ubi nil expurgatur, nec se expedit pulmo, sed propter multitudinem (sputi) fervet in gutture. *Ibid.* 92.

§ CCLXV. At in omnibus pulmonis inflammationibus, si inter initia morbi sputum excernitur flavum, non multò permixtum sanguine, salutare est, & confert admodùm. *Ibid.* 95.

§ CCLXVI. Septimo verò die ac tardiùs, non adeò securum. *Prog.* 96.

§ CCLXVII. Pleuritides graviores sunt quæ sine divulsionibus, quam quæ cùm divulsionibus contingunt. *Coac.* 382.

§ CCLXVIII. Admodùm autem sanguinolentum, aut quod statim ab initio livescit, perniciem præsefert. *Coac.* 390.

§ CCLXIX. Mucosa autem & fuliginosa, tum celeriter colorantur, tum securiora sunt. *Coac. ibid.*

§ CCLXX.

§ CCLXX. Pectora rubris maculis
superfparfa, talibus (fcilicet pleuriticis)
mortem fubeffe teftantur. *Coac.* 417.

§ CCLXXI. Omnia autem fputa mala
funt quæ dolorem non fedant. Optima
quæ fedant. *Præn.* 97, 98.

§ CCLXXII. In morbo laterali, quibus
circa initia in totum purulenta funt fputa,
ii tertiâ die moriuntur. Quos fi fuperent,
nec longè meliùs habuerint, feptimo,
aut nono, aut undecimo fuppurati fiúnt.
Coac. 379.

§ CCLXXIII. A peripneumoniâ phre-
nitis, malum. *Aph.* VII. 12.

§ CCLXXIV. Qui pleuritide laborant,
nifi intra dies 14, fuperne repurgentur,
iis in empyema (id eft in fuppurationem)
fit mali tranflatio. *Aph.* V. 8.

§ CCLXXV. Horum verò locorum dolores qui neque per fputorum purgatio-
nes, neque fæcum alvi dejectionem, ne-

L l   que

que venæfectionem, aut medicamenta purgantia & victûs rationem fedantur: eos ad fuppurationem tendere fciendum eft. *Præn.* 99.

§ CCLXXVI. Suppurationis autem initium fore ratione comprehendere oportet, ab eo die quo primùm æger febricitavit, aut etiam primùm rigor prehendit, & fi pro dolore fibi pondus ineffe in eo loco qui dolore affligebatur, dixerit. Ifta namque circa fuppurationum initia fieri folent. Ex hoc igitur tempore fuppurationum ruptionem fore intrà prædicta tempora expectandum eft. *Ibid.* 103.

§ CCLXXVII. Quibus morbo defunctis horrores crebro cientur, iis pro hæmorrhagiâ fit empyema, id eft fuppuratio. *Coac.* 16.

§ CCLXXVIII. Lateris dolor cum febre diuturnâ, pus eductum iri fignificat. *Coac.* 421.

§ CCLXXIX.

§ CCLXXIX. Qui perhorrefcunt crebro, ad fuppurationem deveniunt. *Ibid.*
422.

§ CCLXXX. Qui ex morbo laterali
faftidiofi fiunt, exudantes, cardialgici,
cum facie rubicundâ & alvo liquidâ:
iis fuppurationes fiunt in pulmone.
Ibid. 423.

§ CCLXXXI. Quod fi in altero tantùm
latere fuppuratio fuerit: tum vertere,
tum edifcere ad hæc convenit, num dolor
aliquis alterum latus detineat, & num
altero calidius fuerit, atque ubi in latus
fanum decubuerit, interrogare, fi quod
ei pondus defuper impendere videatur.
Sic enim altero latere in quo pondus extiterit, fuppuratio eft. *Præn.* 104.

§ CCLXXXII. At purulentos omnes
his fignis dignofcere oportet. Primùm
quidem fi febris non dimittit, verùm interdiù levior quidem, noctu verò major
detinet. Et fudores multis oboriuntur,
tuffefque & tuffiendi cupiditas ipfis ineft,

nihil

nihil tamen effatu dignum expuunt : ocu-
lique cavi redduntur, malæ ruborem con-
trahunt, & ungues quidem in manibus
adunci fiunt, digiti verò, maximèque
fummi incalefcunt, & in pedibus tumores
fiunt, cibos minimè appetunt, & puſtulæ
toto corpore oriuntur. *Præn.* 105.

§ CCLXXXIII. Raucitas cum tuſſi
& alvo liquidâ, pus educit. *Coac.* 414.

§ CCLXXXIV. Diuturnæ igitur fuppurationes his indicantur fignis, quibus
multa fides habenda eſt. Quæ verò bre-
ve habent fpatium, fic indicantur : fi
quid eorum appareant, quæ inter initia
fiunt, fimulque fi etiam aliquanto difficiliùs fpiret æger. *Præn.* 106.

§ CCLXXXV. Ex fuppurationibus autem admodùm exitiales funt, quæ fputo
adhuc quidem biliofo exiſtente fuppurantur, five biliofum illud feparatim, five
unà cum pure expuatur. Idque potiſſi-
mùm, fi ab hujufmodi fputo fuppuratio
procedere cœperit, cum morbus ad diem
feptimum

feptimum pervenerit; qui verò talia fpu‐
it, ne decimo-quarto die moriatur metus‐
eft, nifi quid boni accefferit. *Ibid.* 100.

§ CCLXXXVI. Aᴛ in bonis quidem
fignis hæc numerantur: facilè morbum
fuftinere, benè fpirare, dolore levari, fpu‐
tum fine difficultate rejicere, corpus æ‐
qualiter calidum & molle videri, fine fiti
effe; urinas etiam, & alvi excrementa,
& fomnos, & fudores, veluti defcriptum
eft, fingula fupervenire, bona exiftimanda
funt. His enim omnibus fic contingen‐
tibus, haud quaquam æger morietur.
Quod fi ex his quædam quidem contin‐
gant, quædam minimè, non ultrà deci‐
mum-quartum diem æger vitam produ‐
cet. *Ibid.* 101.

§ CCLXXXVII. Coɴᴛʀᴀ verò, mor‐
bum ægre fuftinere, fpirationem mag‐
nam & denfam effe, dolorem minimè fe‐
dari, fputum ægre rejicere, vehementem
fitim effe, corpus à febre inæqualiter de‐
tineri, alvum quidem, & latera vehemen‐
ter calere, fronte, manibus & pedibus
frigidis;

frigidis; urinas verò, & alvi excrementa,
& somnos, & sudores, unaquæque qualia
descripta sunt, mala esse nosse convenit.
Si quid enim ex his sputo supervenerit,
morietur æger, priusquam ad decimum-
quartum diem perveniat, aut nono, aut
undecimo die. Sic igitur conjicere oportet, quod cum sputum istud valde lethale
sit, neque etiam ad decimum-quartum
diem perducit. Ex his verò, tum malo-
rum, tum bonorum subductâ ratione,
prædictiones facere oportet, sic enim quis
potissimum verum assequatur. *Ibid.* 102.

§ CCLXXXVIII. Reliquæ verò suppurationes, magnâ ex parte rumpuntur,
partìm quidem vigesimo die, partìm etiam trigesimo, quædam quoque quadra-
gesimo, aliquæ etiam ad sexagesimum
diem deveniunt. *Ibid.* 102.

§ CCLXXXIX. At ex his quæ citiùs,
aut tardiùs rumpuntur, sic deprehendere
licet. Siquidem dolor inter initia oriatur,
& spirandi difficultas, ac tussis sputatio-
que perseverant, & ad vigesimum diem
exten-

extenduntur: intra hoc tempus, aut adhuc prius ruptionem expectato. Quod
si mitior dolor fuerit, iisque cætera omnia pro hujus ratione respondeant, tardius raptionem sperato. *Ibid.* 107.

§ CCXC. At antè puris eruptionem,
dolorem oboriri, & spirandi difficultatem,
& sputi excretionem, necesse est. *Ibid.*

§ CCXCI. Supersunt autem ex morbo hi potissimum, quos febris eodem post
ruptionem die dimisit, quique cibos celeriter expetiverint, & siti liberantur, ven-
terque tum exigua, tum coacta dejicit,
& si pus album & læve, ejusdemque coloris fuerit, & à pituitâ liberum, citraque
dolorem, aut tussim vehementem educa-
tur. Sic quidem optimè, & celerrimè
liberantur: sin minùs, qui ad ista proximè
accedent. *Ibid.* 108.

§ CCXCII. Moriuntur verò, quos
febris non dimiserit, aut cum dimisisse
videatur, iterum accenditur, & siti quidem vexantur, cibos verò non expetiverint;

rint; & fi alvus liquida dejecerit, pufque
ex viridi pallidum, aut pituitâ permixtum, & fpumofum expuerint. Si hæc
omnia contigerint, moriuntur. *Ibid.* 109.

§ CCXCIII. A⊤ quibus eorum partìm
quædam contigerint, partìm minimè, ex
his non nulli quidem intereunt, quidam
etiam ex longo temporis intervallo fuper-
funt. Sed ex omnibus his fignis exiften-
tibus, tum in his, tum in relɪquis omnibus, conjecturam facito. *Ibid.* 110.

§ CCXCIV. Ex iis verò qui à pulmonis inflammationibus fuppurantur, ferè
feniores moriuntur, at ex cæteris fuppurationibus juniores potiùs intereunt.
Ibid. 117.

§ CCXCV. Qui ex pleuritide empyi
fiunt (*id eft purulenti, abfceffu laborantes*)
fi à ruptione intra dies quadraginta fursùm purgenter, liberantur. Alioqui tran-
feunt in tabem. *Aph.* V. 15.

§ CCXCVI.

§ CCXCVI. Quibus purulentis mitiora fiunt omnia, si posteà pus edunt foedi odoris, iis recidiva mortifera. *Coac.* 406.

§ CCXCVII. Ex tuberculi intùs ruptione exolutio, vomitus & animi deliquium fit. *Aph.* VII. 8.

. § CCXCVIII. Cum suppurati uruntur, si purum pus fuerit, & album, nec tetri odoris, convalescunt. At quibus subcruentum, & cænosum, moriuntur. *Præn.* 119.

§ CCXCIX. Quibus concutiendo pus editur cænosum, & foedi odoris, ut plurimùm moriuntur. *Coac.* 409.

§ CCC. Quibus à pure coloratur specillum tanquam ab igne, maximam illi partem intereunt. *Coac.* 410.

§ CCCI. Quibus intumuit latus, ac incaluit, si cum in oppositam partem decumbunt grave quidpiam suspensum esse

videatur,

videatur, pus ab unâ parte colleꞔum eſt.
Ibid. 428.

§ CCCII. Inter empyicos, quibus con-
cuſſis humeris multus fit ſtrepitus, parci-
ùs illi pus habent, quam quibus exiguus,
modò ſpirent faciliùs, & meliùs ſint colo-
rati. At quibus ne minimus quidem in-
fertur, ſed fortis diſpnæe lividique ungues, pleni ſunt illi pure, ac deſperati.
Ibid. 432.

De Anginâ.

§ CCCIII. Angina graviſſima quidem
eſt & celerrimè interimit quæ neque in
faucibus, nec in cervice quicquam conſpi-
cuum facit; plurimùm verò doloris exhibet, & difficultatem ſpirandi quæ ereꞔâ
cervice obitur inducit. Hæc enim eodem
etiam die, & ſecundo, & tertio, & quarto
ſtrangulat. *Præn.* 132.

§ CCCIV. Quibus Anginâ liberatis ad
pulmonem mali fit converſio, ii intra ſeptem

tem dies moriuntur, quos si effugerint, suppurati evadunt. *Aph.* V. 10.

De sputo sanguinis & phtyseos periculo.

§ CCCV. Tabes maximè fit ab anno octavo-decimo, ad trigesimum-quintum.. *Aph.* V. 9.

§ CCCVI. A sanguinis sputo puris sputum, à puris sputo tabes, à tabe, mors.

§ CCCVII. Qui sanguinem evomunt, si sine febre salutare, si cum febre, malum. *Aph.* VII. 37.

§ CCCVIII. Qui sanguinem evomunt spumantem, omnique dolore carent sub diaphragmate, à pulmone vomunt. Et quibus in ipso rupta est magna vena, multum illi vomunt, & periculosè admodùm: & quibus minor, minùs rejiciunt, & securiores sunt. *Coac.* 433.

M m 2 § CCCIX.

§ CCCIX. In metu funt maximo phty-
fes, quæ à ruptione venarum craffarum,
aut à catarrho è capite contingunt. *Coac.*
438.

Circà apoplexiam.

§ CCCX. Apoplectici fiunt maximè
à quadragefimo anno ad fexagefimum.
Aph. VI. 57.

§ CCCXI. Qui naturâ funt valdè craffi,
magis fubitò moriuntur, quàm graciles.
Aph. II. 44.

§ CCCXII. Torpores & ftupores præter confuetudinem evenientes, futura denunciant apoplectica. *Coac.* 476.

§ CCCXIII. Quibus febre vacuis ce-
phalagia, tinnitus aurium, unàque tene-
bricofa vertigo incidit, & vocis tarditas,
& manuum ftupor : his vcl apoplexia, vel
epilepfia, aut lethargus imminet. *Coac.*
161.

§ CCCXIV.

§ CCCXIV. Qui valentes, capitis repentè doloribus corripiuntur, & protinùs muti fiunt, & ftertunt, intrà dies feptem intereunt, nifi febris eos prehenderit. *Aph.* VI. 51.

§ CCCXV. Solvere apoplexiam fortem impoffibile, levem difficile. *Aph.* II. 42.

§ CCCXVI. In apoplecticis ex magna refpirandi difficultate fubortus fudor, mortem affert. *Coac.* 479.

N O T E S.

N O T E S.

---

§ II. (* 1.)

WE can hardly flatter ourselves, that the Phyficians of different countries, will ever agree, in giving, conftantly, the fame names to the fame fevers. But, although they may differ as to thefe nominal diftinctions, it is effential for them, to agree with, and underftand each other, as to the things themfelves. To this purpofe, it is neceffary for them, to defcribe, with accuracy and precifion, the fevers they mean to indicate, under fuch and fuch a denomination. I have fpoken in another work of malignant fevers (a). In that performance, I aimed at carefully and clearly pointing out the fevers, to which the French phyficians are accuftomed to give the name of *malignant*. It will not

---

(a) *Memoires fur les fievres aiguës.*

be

be amifs, I believe, here, again to explain and illuf-
trate, and even, in fome refpects, to rectify my ideas
on this fubject; as well for the information of young
phyficians, as of foreigners, who may happen to read
this work; and who, without fuch an explanation,
might perhaps, have fome doubts, of the nature of
the acute fevers, to which I have fo often applied
the epithet of *malignant,* in the courfe of my obfervations.

After attentive confideration, of all that I have
feen and read, on the fubject of acute continued
fevers, I am of opinion, that thefe difeafes may be
very properly diftributed into two general claffes.
The firft of thefe, I ftile Inflammatory, and the
fecond, Malignant Fevers. Thefe two claffes are
diftinguifhed from each other by the following
figns. In the courfe of inflammatory fevers, the *vis
vitæ* feems to be augmented inftead of being weakened. The pulfe is ufually open and expanded,
(etendu, developpé); fometimes, however, it is fmall;
but, in both cafes, has a degree of ftrength Thefe
fevers readily fupport blood-letting. The heat of
the body, the thirft, head-ach, delirium, difficulty of
breathing, and, in a word, all the fymptoms that
are liable to take place, are proportioned nearly to
the violence of fever, to the frequency, ftrength,
and hardnefs of the pulfe. Thefe fevers do not
fuddenly deftroy the animal powers. If the pulfe
becomes foft and weak; either this fymptom is dependent only on fome tranfitory caufe, and, in that
cafe, does not laft long; or, it is, becaufe life begins
to be extinguifhed from an irremediable affection of
fome of the vifcera. To this clafs, I refer pleurify,
and other fymptomatic inflammatory fevers, and
likewife

likewife eruptive fevers, and laftly, the other continued fevers, that afford the figns I have defcribed.'

Malignant fevers feem to attack, at once, the principle of life. From their very beginning, both the
animal and vital powers appear to be weakened.
The pulfe is weak and foft, and almoft always fmall,
depreffed, and fometimes irregular. The fymptoms
are not always proportioned to the degree of fever.
The delirium, coma, difficulty of breathing, tumefaction of the abdomen, pains, inflammatory fwelling of the hypochondria, convulfions, and other
dangerous fymptoms, ufually occur in thefe fevers,
although the pulfe remains fmall, funk, foft, and
weak. Venæfection, efpecially if repeated, feems to
diminifh the ftrength of the patient, and to do harm
inftead of relieving him.

Such are the figns, which feem to me to belong
the moft generally to fevers of this clafs; and which
may likewife be diftinguifhed by many other fymptoms, that are not obferved in inflammatory fevers.
Thus the onfet of a malignant fever, is ufually characterized by naufea, or by fatiguing and obftinate
vomiting; acute pains in the loins, thighs, and legs.
In their progrefs, they likewife afford fwelling of the
face, deafnefs, fubfultus tendinum, buboes, carbuncles, &c. purple fpots, vibices, &c. gangrenous
eryfipelas, and other fymptoms, which fufficiently
denote and confirm the character of malignancy.
Malignant fevers do likewife, very often, leave fatal
impreffions on the origin of the nerves. Of the
patients who efcape with life, we fee fome remain
a long time deaf, or deprived of fight; and others,

who

who have loft their memory, or judgment, or who have an infenfibility of fome of their limbs. Fevers, of this fort, are alfo generally, though not always contagious, and are much more deftructive than thofe of the inflammatory clafs.

Phyficians are nearly agreed, as to the epidemic acute fevers. which belong to the clafs of malignant fevers. They almoft all concur in arranging together under this head, plague, peftilential fevers, purple malignant fevers, petechial fevers (b), and exanthematic catarrhal fevers (c). The fevers, produced by the infectious air of fhips, prifons, and hofpita's are likewife evidently to be referred to the fame clafs (d) The improper conftruction of our prifons, has afforded me frequent opportunities of obferving the different epidemical fevers, that are the refult of infectious air. This matter is fufficiently illuftrated by Dr. Lind, in his paper on fevers and infections; and by Sir John Pringle, in his excellent defcription of the jail fever. Although that celebrated writer does not defcribe it under the name of malignant fever, yet it is not the lefs

---

(b) F Hoffman Med Rat. Tom. II. p. 84.

(c) Ibid. p. 84. *Febris catarrhalis maligna petechizans.*

(d) The celebrated Dr. Cullen has very properly confidered all the feveral kinds of fever here mentioned, the plague excepted, as fo many fynonyma, rather than varieties, of Typhus, which he defines, " Morbus contagiofus, calor parum auctus; " pulfus parvus, debilis, plerumque frequens; fenforii func- " tiones plurimum turbatæ; vires multum imminutæ".—The plague he has very judicioufly arranged, in the order of exanthemata, as being typhus, attended with an eruption of bubo or carbuncle. See his *Synopf. Nofol. Method. pag.* 287.

clear,

clear, that he thinks as we do, as to its real nature. " It is evident," fays he, " that this diftemper is of " a truly peftilential nature, as appears by the man- " ner in which the head is affected, by the dejection " of the fpirits, debility, funk pulfe, the fuppu- " ration of the parotid and axillary glands, the pu- " trid fweats, petechial fpots, mortifications, and " contagion (e).

On confidering the numerous defcriptions of epi- demical fevers, of this clafs, that are to be met with in authors, and of feveral others of the fame kind, on account of which, the faculty at Montpelier has been confulted within thefe twelve years, it feems evident, that thefe fevers differ from each other by an infinity of fhades. Experience proves, that even epidemical fevers, of the fame feafon, differ from each other, and undergo wonderful changes in the eyes of attentive obfervers. Fevers for example, that are at firft very contagious, rapid in their pro- grefs, and deftructive, at length appear with more mo- deration, and, becoming lefs fatal, no longer afford the fame fymptoms they did at the beginning of the epidemic (f). All thefe epidemical fevers prefer- ving, therefore, a remarkable analogy to each other, by the lofs of ftrength, by the ftate of the pulfe, by the

---

(e) Obfervations on the Difeafes of the Army, p 319, 6th edit. 8vo.

(f) Every epidemic paffes, by an almoft infenfible gradation, through its feveral periods of rife, acmé, and decline. All accu- rate obfervations, from the time of Hippocrates downwards, prove this; but yet the diftinguifhing character of the difeafe continues the fame, though it may vary in violence, from the difference of feafon, and occur with different fymptoms,

according

the bad effects of blood-letting, and by the eruptions and other symptoms that are familiar to them,
differ, however, very considerably from each other,
by their progrefs and duration, and by their degree
of contagion; or, by fome fymptom or eruption,
that is peculiar to fome one or more of them, without
being common to all. Thefe varieties are fo numerous, that it feems to me to be impoffible to inform
onefelf, fufficiently, of the true nature of each, by
any other means, than by attentive obfervation,
united to the beft defcriptions in this way, that are to
be met with in authors. They, who with Sennertus,
have included, and defcribed them all, under the
name of plague, or peftilential, or malignant fevers;
or, with Hoffman, under the name of peftilential (g)
fever, true petechial fever, and epidemic catarrhal

---

according to the various predifpofition of different fubjects.
The great Sydenham very aptly remarks, that " how many
" peculiar fpecies foever arife in one and the fame conftitu-
" tion, they all agree in being produced by one common ge-
" neral caufe, viz. fome peculiar ftate of the air; and, con-
" fequently, how much foever they may differ fiom one ano-
" ther in appearance, and fpecific nature, yet, the conftitu-
" tion, common to them all, works upon the fubject matter
" of each, and moulds it to fuch a ftate and condition, that
" the principal fymptoms (provided they have no regard to
" the particular manner of evacuation) are alike in all; all of
" them agreeing in this circumftance, that they refpectively
" grow mild or violent at the fame time. It is further to be
" noted, that in whatever years thefe feveral fpecies prevail, at
" one and the fame time, the fymptoms wherewith they
" come on, are alike in all." *Swan's edit. page* 9.

(g) The epithet ' peftilential', feems to have been very
often liberally applied, by writers, to fevers that were not contagious, when they were epidemical and deftructive.

exanthematous

exanthematous fever, or, *febris catarrhalis petechizans*; may, indeed, be said to have caught some of the moſt ſtriking ſhades of thoſe fevers; but they are far (or I am deceived) fiom affording us preciſe ideas of all the extent of this claſs of diſeaſes, and from giving their readers a previous notion of all the variety they may expect in them.

If I am now aſked, what are the ſporadic fevers, to which the Fiench phyſicians give the epithet of malignant; I am diſpoſed to anſwer, that they are preciſely the ſporadic fevers, which afford evident analogy to the epidemical fevers we have juſt now mentioned. Let us ſuppoſe, for inſtance, that three or four French phyſicians viſit a patient, and diſtinguiſh his diſorder by the name of putrid fever, and that, there afterwards comes on ſubſultus tendinum, or deafneſs, or ſuppuration of the parotid glands, or ſome of the other ſymptoms, that are familiar to peſtilential and malignant epidemical fevers; they will then ſay, that the nature of the diſeaſe is altered, and that it has degenerated into a malignant fever: or, if they are men of candour, they will freely own, that it has always been of the malignant kind, but that they were miſtaken in the beginning.

It is, therefore, on their reſemblance to epidemical, peſtilential, and malignant fevers, that phyſicians, in France, eſtabliſh their notions of malignant ſporadic fevers. The leaſt inſtructed of them, are acquainted only with a few of the points of analogy, theſe two kinds of fever afford; ſuch as ſwellings of the parotid glands, purple ſpots, deafneſs, ſubſultus tendinum, carbuncle, or ſome other ſymptom.

equally

equally manifeft. It therefore often happens, that the nature of thefe malignant fporadic fevers, is not fufficiently known, until their danger is become evident even to the by-ftanders. Such miftakes can be avoided only by ftudying, with minute and fcrupulous attention, all the fymptoms that are common to malignant fevers, whether epidemic or fporadic.

Our cuftom of charaéterizing, as malignant fevers, every fporadic fever, that affords a remarkable analogy to peftilential epidemical fevers, takes its fource from the moft refpeétable authors. I have, in another place *(h)*, obferved, that Galen acknowledged the exiftence of fporadic peftilential fevers, that is, of fevers, which attacking only individuals, afford, however, the fame fymptoms as epidemical peftilential fevers. Many writers have adopted this opinion of Galen's; and Fernelius having given to them the name of malignant fevers, it is likely, that the authority of fo refpeétable a name, has gradually eftablifhed the ufe of this denomination in France. It feems probable too, that the authority of Sydenham *(i)* has prevented the Englifh from adopting it.

I fhall

(h) Memoires fur les fievres aiguës.

(i) " *The invention of the term, or opinion of malignity,*—fays " that truly great man—*has been far more deftruétive to mankind,* " *than the ufe of gun-powder.*" Dr. Huxham, however, is of a different opinion, and fpeaking on this fubjeét, fays, " I am " very fenfible, the word *malignant* as applied to fevers, hath " of late years, fallen into very great difrepute, and probably " it hath been often made ufe of to cover ignorance, or magni- " fy a cure.—But there is, really, a foundation in nature, for " fuch

['279]

I fhall add nothing here, to what I have already faid in the Memoirs I refer to, on the different kinds of fporadic malignant fevers. But I ought not to conclude this note, without citing what I have advanced in the third fection of the fecond part of that work: where I fay, " It is doubtlefs better, " and more agreeable to the ftile of obfervation, " to give a general idea of thefe fevers, by an

---

" fuch an appellation, at leaft, for fome word that may diftin-
" guifh fuch a difeafe, as I have been now defcribing, (putrid
" malignant fever) from a common inflammatory fever, indeed
" the very term, *inflammatory fever*, fuppofes there are other
" kinds of fevers.—It is, perhaps, indifferent, whether you call
" them putrid, malignant, or peftilential: when petechiæ ap-
" pears, every one calls them fpotted, or petechial; and if from
" contagion, contagious   I will contend with nobody about
" words, but it is neceffary we fhould have fome to communi-
" cate our ideas, and where they are well defined, no one hath
" great reafon to quarrel with them " Effay on fevers, page
101.   It will not be amifs, to hear what M Sauvages fays on
this head   In his Nofology, we find *continued malignant fever,
nervous fever*, and the *Typhodes of Profper Alpini*, ufed as the
fynonyma of Typhus, which is the name of the Genus, adopted
from Hippocrates and which Dr. Cullen has likewife introduced in his arrangement.   " It is called malignant," fays M.
de Sauvages, " becaufe it brings the patients fecretly into dan-
" ger, the heat, the pulfe, and the urine, appearing as in the
" healthy ftate; and likewife, becaufe it fuddenly brings on the
" moft alarming fymptoms, fuch as dejection of fpirits, deliri-
" um, cardialgia, exanthema, and convulfions; altho' at the
" beginning, it feemed to threaten no danger.   I am aware,
" that in France, phyficians in general, ftile all fevers malig-
" nant. that are accompanied with any dangerous and extraor-
" dinary fymptoms · but there are others who pretend, that this
" term is applicable only to the fevers arifing from contagious,
" or venomous miafmata, to avoid all equivocations, we may
" apply the word *Typhus*, to the genus, and leave the epithet
" of *malignant* to its fpecies." *Nofol. Method*   Tom. 1.
                                        " enumeration

" enumeration of the symptoms that are familiar
" to, and help to distinguish them; such as the
" obstinate vomiting, the subsultus tendinum, the
" weakness and irregularity of the pulse, &c. or,
" if a shorter definition is required, they may be
" stiled dangerous and destructive fevers." The
observations I have made, since the publication of
that work, have convinced me, that I ought to
have confined myself to the first part of this asser-
tion, and to have contented myself, with observing, that of the acute continued essential fevers,
(*fievres continuès aiguès essentielles*) the only ones
treated of in those Memoirs, there are some, which,
although of an inflammatory nature, and affording none of the symptoms familiar to malignant
fevers, bring, however, the patients into the
greatest danger. But, I believe, I do not say too
much, when I assert, that for one acute essential
fever of this sort. which will carry off a patient,
we shall observe twenty similar terminations, the
result of malignant fevers.

Independent of fevers, properly so called, there
are other Acute Diseases, which sometimes partake of the nature of malignant fevers; and
which, it will be necessary, to distinguish, by a
name, that may sufficiently characterize them.
Such are evidently, the gangrenous sore throat,
and certain pleurisies, dysenteries, and some kinds
of small pox; for all these diseases, may be properly stiled malignant, whenever the extreme re-
duction of the patient's strength, the state of the
pulse, the bad effects of bleeding, especially, of
repeated bleeding. and purple spots, or other
symptoms,

fymptoms, denote the analogy or affinity ; or, if you will, an evident complication, with the deſtructive fevers, known and deſcribed under the names of peſtilential or malignant fevers.

§ III. (* 2.)

Such is the uſual progreſs of acute fevers ; even of thoſe, in the courſe of which, the pulſe has the moſt ſtrength   When a diſeaſe, that is purely inflammatory, or a deep wound, or a compound fracture, terminate in death, the pulſe, from being ſtrong, becomes ſmall, ſoft, weak, and often irregular, and continues ſo. This obſervation may be extended ſtill farther, and will be found to hold good, even in chronic diſeaſes. Whenever the ſtrength of a patient ſeems exhauſted by a diſeaſe of this ſort, and his pulſe aſſumes and preſerves the character we have juſt now mentioned, we may be aſſured, that his death is not far diſtant. It uſually happens within a week, ſeldom later than a fortnight, after ſuch a change has taken place.

§ V. (3.)

To form a ſound judgment of the ſtate of the pulſe, it will be right to apply our fingers to the artery with different degrees of preſſure. If the pulſe has really much ſtrength, the pulſation will be ſelt more ſmartly, in proportion as we preſs upon the artery ; whereas, if it be weak, it will

be

be felt lefs and lefs, and at length will feem to
be altogether extinguifhed, as we increafe the
preffure.

§ XIV. (* 4)

When this happens, we are to confider, whether the fever, that affords fuch a fymptom, is of
the clafs of intermittents or continued fevers; becaufe fyncope will, in general, be lefs alarming
in the former than in the latter; and we fhall
have greater hopes of being able to prevent its
return, by means of the bark.

§ XV. (* 5.)

On opening the bodies of thofe who have died,
and who have experienced this fymptom towards
the clofe of the difeafe, the inteftines have ufually
been found white and tranfparent, fo much have
they been diftended with air.

§ XXXIX. (* 6.)

The pains of the breaft, in this cafe, are lefs fixed and lafting, than when occafioned by a true affection of the breaft. The cough that accompanies
them, is dry. It is not conftant, and fometimes occurs only during the exacerbations. See § LXI.

§ LIV.

§ LIV. (* 7.)

Diſſections prove, that a ſerous effuſion into the cavity of the abdomen, or thorax, is a pretty common effect of a fatal inflammation of the viſcera of either of thoſe cavities. See § xxxi.

§ LIX. (* 8.)

Such, in my opinion, is the reſult of obſervations. If I inquire after the reaſon, it ſeems to me, to be found in the expectoration, which we know to be the great reſource of nature, in inflammations of the breaſt. We know of no evacuation, that is ſo familiar to her, and, at the ſame time, ſo generally deciſive, in inflammations of the abdominal viſcera.

§ LXXX. (* 9.)

It is to this ſort of delirium, we may apply the expreſſion of Fernelius, *Majoris terroris eſt quam periculi* (*k*). It would very often be contrary to truth, if applied to every kind of delirium.

§ LXXXII. (* 10.)

Qui ſuprà quadraginta annos phrentici fiunt,—ſays Hippocrates—*non ad modum ſanantur.* This parti-

---

(*k*) *De febr. cap.* 19.

culax

cular obfervation is, without doubt, one of thofe, which led him to eftablifh the following general pro-pofition : *in morbis minùs periclitantur quorum naturæ, ætati, et temperamento, et tempeſtati magis affinis fue-rit morbus, quàm in quibus horum nulli fuerit affinis.* Aphorifm, 11. § xxiv. The reader will have re-marked in the courfe of this work, that this affertion of Hippocrates, may be very properly applied to a great number of Acute Difeafes. I have not thought it right to employ the above aphorifm, becaufe, be-ing too general, it admits of many exceptions, efpe-cially in chronic difeafes.

§ XC. (* 11.)

Qui ad manum exiliunt, in malo funt. Coac. 75. The commentary of *Duretus* on this paffage of Hippocrates, is not well underftood. Houlier's is clear. He applies this expreffion, *qui ad manus exili-unt*, to fubfultus tendinum. I confefs myfelf, how-ever, to be of opinion, that obfervation leads us to a much more natural explanation of this Prognoftic. Amongft the great variety of delirious patients, we fee fome who are timid, and exceffively fenfible ; and who, in the midft of their diftraction, and when employed on the objects of their delirium, if the phyfician puts his hand on theirs, draw it haftily away, and with marks of fear, as if they aimed at avoiding him. Would it not feem, therefore, as if Hippocrates, by the words, *qui ad manum exilunt*, alluded to this fymptom, which is a much more natural application, than that of fubfultus tendinum. Altho' it may be be of little confequence to afcertain

the

the true meaning of this Prognoftic, yet it is right to know, that the danger of delirium, is conftantly increafed by its being complicated with fubfultus tendinum'; and that delirium, attended with exceffive fenfibility, and timidity, at the leaft touch or noife, is ftill more alarming.

§ CXI.　(* 12.)

Some phyficians will, without doubt, be furprifed to fee me affert, that certain wounds, and fractures, are capable of exciting fevers, which will have fome affinity with malignant fevers. I requeft them to obferve, that I found not the idea, I give of thefe fevers, on any opinion that relates to the caufes, by which they are produced, but wholly on the fymptoms they afford, and which I have enumerated (* 1) And fince we know, that certain wounds, and compound fractures, give rife to fevers, which afford fimilar fymptoms, I fee no reafon why we fhould deny, that thefe fevers, tho' produced by external caufes, are, however, of the fame kind as malignant fevers, and have a remarkable analogy, and affinity with them. A waggon paffes over the leg of an old man, he is carried to bed, and his leg is examined The furgeon raifes it by the foot, but it affords no crepitas, or marks of fracture. A fever, however, begins to appear the fame day, and foon affords the moft alarming fymptoms. The pulfe becomes fmall, foft, weak, and very quick, and the patient is delirious, or comatofe. The phyficians afcribe thefe fymptoms to a malignant fever, produced by the fright. Still, however, as the difeafe increafes

creafes in danger, the contufed leg affords marks of gangrene. The patient dies on the fixth day. On examining the dead body, it is difcovered, that if inftead of raifing the leg by the foot, the furgeon had taken it up by the knee, the fracture would have been eafily felt, as the leg would then have bent ; the ends of the fractured bone, which fupported each other in the firft pofition, being unable to do fo in the other. The diffection of the leg proves too, that the tibia was fractured, and that fome fplinters of the bone had excited the fever and gangrene, and the other fymptoms, that ended in death.

§ CXVII. (* 13)

The epileptic convulfions, that come on towards the clofe of Acute Difeafes, are fometimes preceded by a fenfation of tenfion, in the mufcles of the neck, and by a pain in the throat, that is accompanied, however, neither by rednefs, nor fwelling. A patient, whom I attended, of the name of Agret, was ill of a continued fever. The diforder did not afford any fatal fymptom ; neverthelefs, the patient's countenance, and great weaknefs, alarmed me fo much, that I recommended to his friends, the fettling of his affairs. It was about this time, that he began to complain of a painful tenfion on the right fide of his neck, and of pain in his throat. It was carefully examined by M. Sarraw, his furgeon, and myfelf, but we could difcover no marks of fwelling, or inflammation We had hardly compleated the examination, when the patient was attacked with epileptic convulfions, which were fucceeded by coma,

coma, and death It was, doubtless, the observation of similar cases, that induced Hippocrates to give the following Prognostics. *Fauces valdé dolentes et æquales cum jactatione, crudeliter et cito mortiferæ.* Coac. 265. *Faucium dolor prægrandis parotides et convulsiones facit, atque cervicis et dorsi dolores.* Ibid. 268.

§ CXVII. (* 14.)

Every physician, who has any practice, must necessarily have frequent occasions of being convinced of the propriety of these Prognostics, which are an exception to the doctrine of Hippocrates, *Coac.* 109. that convulsions, in these fevers, are less dangerous when they occur in children under seven years of age. If a physician, who visits a patient so affected, under that age, and should, on the testimony of Hippocrates, take upon him to say, that they are not very dangerous, he would, in my opinion, give as great a proof of his inexperience, as of his erudition.

§ CXXIII. (* 15)

They, who attend women in labour have the most frequent opportunities of observing the truth of this Prognostic When the labour is exceedingly tedious, and painful, it very commonly occasions epileptic convulsions, which, when they are to terminate in death, end in an apoplectic comatose affection. We likewise see, tho' much more rarely,

other

other acute, and long continued pains, exciting convulsions, apoplectic sleep, and death. I suspect it is, to this sort of death, Hippocrates alludes, when he says, *qui ex dolore fuint aphoni, crudeliter moriuntur.* *Coac.* 249.

§ CXLIII. (* 16.)

I give the name of cross palsy, to that kind of hemiplegia, in which the left leg and right arm, or the left arm and right leg are affected. This kind of hemiplegia, is, indeed, very rare, but we sometimes see it happen,

§ CLXIII. (* 17.)

The atrabilious vomiting, is of a deep brown, or blackish colour, not unlike that of soot, when wet with water. This sort of vomiting, when it takes place in Acute Diseases, is fatal: in chronic diseases, it likewise denotes the patient to be near his end. We are to be careful, however, not to attach so unfavourable an idea to it, when it occurs in a fit of atrabilious colic. I will, therefore, observe here, as a caution to young physicians, that there are persons, who, from a peculiarity of temperament, or by habitual errors in diet, have a matter of this sort continually forming, and that this, when accumulated to a certain degree, brings on a fit of colic. The paroxysms are characterized by the vomiting of a brown, blackish matter, usually of an exceedingly acrid and sometimes very rancid, taste. The duration

ration of the fit is of confiderable variety In fome
it is over in a few hours ; in others it lafts feven or
eight hours, without producing any fatal effects. I
have a patient, in whom I have had occafion to fee
more than thirty of thefe paroxyfms, in the fpace
of eight and twenty years.

§ CLXVI. (* 18.)

The iliac paffion, an Acute Difeafe, is characterized by the following figns. Nothing paffes downwards. The patient is almoft inceffantly vomiting.
Every time he pukes, he finds himfelf relieved, but,
this relief is of fhort duration. Thirft foon obliges
him to drink. The naufea begins again, and the
vomiting. The matter he brings up, is of various colours, yellow, green, &c. All, however,
agree in depofiting a fort of minced matter, a kind
of grounds. Towards the clofe of the difeafe,
when it ends in death, the matter thus thrown up,
diffufes, commonly, a fœtid, ftercoral odor.

Sometimes the patients vomit up entire portions
of excrement. This, however, does not often happen. The generality of thofe who perifh by this
cruel difeafe, commonly dying without having any
vomiting of this fort. An acute fever is always complicated with this diforder, when it is of fhort duration. The rapidity of its progrefs, is proportioned
to the violence of its fymptoms. If the fever is
acute, as well as the pain, and the vomiting, and
diftrefs afford the patient no interval of repofe, it
ufually terminates in a few days. Sometimes it runs

on

on to the tenth, fifteenth, and even thirtieth day, when the fymptoms are moderate.

If it be effential to define difeafes, and to characterize them by the figns they afford in their very beginning, it would certainly be erroneous to diftinguifh this by a vomiting of matter that fmells like excrement, becaufe this takes place only towards the clofe of the difeafe, when it ends in death; much lefs fhould we fay vomiting of excrement, becaufe this very feldom takes place at any period of the difeafe. Experience feems to have proved to me, that, independent of the other fymptoms, the iliac vomiting is chiefly characterized by the minced matter, the fort of grounds of which I fpoke.

The accidents, occafioned by ftrangulated hernia, and, likewife, an infinite number of diffections, prove, that the iliac paffion is produced, every time the inteftinal canal is obftructed or compreffed, fo that the free progrefs of the fœces towards the anus, is intercepted. Admitting that the difeafe may take place, merely by an inverfion of the periftaltic motion; and fupporting this argument by what has, fometimes, been feen to happen in the cafes of clyfters, and fuppofitories voided at the mouth, yet it would be to renounce every days experience, in favour of fome few marvellous obfervations, which are the more fufpicious, as not being confirmed by the obfervations of our moft experienced practitioners (l.)

When

(l.) The ancients do not feem to have confidered vomiting as a pathognomonic fymptom of the λειος, ileus. Hippocrates obferves, that εν ω εμετος ληξ και, Aphor Sect. vir which fhews,

When the free paffage of any part of the inteftinal canal, becomes fuddenly and totally intercepted, the difeafe, refulting from it, is an acute iliac paffion, whether it arife from inflammation, introfufception, hernia, a bundle of worms, hardened fœces, or the hufks of grapes, or other fruit, &c. (m).

But

---

fhews, that he thought there might be ileus, without either of thefe.—The moderns, however, feem to agree to give the name of iliac paffion, only when the periftaltic motion is inverted. When this inverfion procceds from hardened excrements, or flatus, or ftrangulated hernia, or tumours within the cavity of the abdomen, or from inflammation, Sydenham will allow the difeale to be only a *fpurious iliac paffion*, becaufe, fays he, it is not, " *an inverfion of the whole duet, but of thofe parts only, which* " *are fituated above the feat of the obftruction.*" He gives the name of *true iliac paffion* to the difeafe, only when the irritation and inverfion of the periftaltic motion extends through the whole of the canal, and this, amongft other figns, " appears " from clyfters being vomited up," a proof that the great man had feen this fymptom take place.

Sir John Pringle fays, he faw this *true ileus* of Sydenham only once, (the patient died) and he imagines that it has been but rarely feen in our times, by thofe in the greateft practice, and feldom or never cured. *Obf. on the Dif. of an Army.*

Boerhaave fpeaking on this fubject, fays, " Teftes funt gra- " viffimi viri, non fcybala fola, fed ipfos aliquando clyfteres " per os ejectes fuiffe, (verum ftercus alvinum ipfe per os excerni " vidi, 1732.") Prælect Academ. de Inftit. Tom. vi. page 204. Other authorities might be quoted, but it is prefumed, that thefe three refpectable ones will be fufficient to prove, that altho' the fymptom in queftion, may not have occurred to the learned author, and is, indeed, a very rare one, yet that it really has fometimes happened.

(m) The reader will meet with feveral interefting cafes of hardened fœces, and of plumb ftones retained in the intef-

tines,

But if the diameter of any part of the inteſtinal canal. is, by any means, gradually diminiſhed, whether it be by primary affection of the inteſtine itſelf, or by the preſſure of ſome neighbouring tumour, there comes on another kind of iliac paſſion, which may be ſtiled a chronic diſeaſe. This chronic iliac paſſion, becomes eſtabliſhed by almoſt inſenſible degrees. In general, the patients begin by feeling a ſort of weight or embarraſſment, in ſome part of the lower belly, and this always, at the ſame place, and at the ſame period, after a meal. They have a diſieliſh, and ſometimes an averſion for food. Sometime after a repaſt their mouth abounds with ſaliva, and they ſpit conſiderably. At length, when the diſeaſe is more eſtabliſhed, they vomit. This vomiting, in general, takes place ſoon after a meal, ſometimes, however, not till long afterwards. The matter, they bring up by vomiting, is aliment, more or leſs digeſted, and ſlimy, bilious matter, varying in its colour, .but which depoſits the ſort of grounds,

---

tines, in a collection of caſes in ſurgery, publiſhed by the ingenious Mr. White, of Mancheſter —There are ſimilar accounts likewiſe, in Philoſ. Tranſ. abridged, vol. v p. 256, et ſeq. Edin. Eſſay, vol. 1. and vol v. and in Eſſays Phyſ. and Literary, vol. ii. Hardened balls, and even ſtoney concretions, are, ſometimes, met with in the colon —The *nucleus* of theſe, is generally a fruit ſtone, ſimilar concretions are more frequent in ſome other animals, eſpecially cows and horſes.—I have taken ſtones of this ſort, from the colon of a horſe, that weighed more than three pounds.—The colon, from its ſtructure, is particularly liable to theſe concretions. The ſeat of the dyſentery is known to be chiefly in this part of the canal, and we are ſenſible how much the irritation is kept up by the hardened fœces in that diſeaſe.

I ſpoke

I fpoke of as characterizing the iliac vomiting. In this cafe, the belly is not completely bound. Clyf- ters, and gentle laxatives, ufually procure ftools. But the difeafe is not the lefs certainly fatal; and when it takes place in a chronic difeafe, we may expect that the patient will inevitably die.

§ CLXXXVI. (* 19.)

Thefe ftools, when they have been preceded, nei- ther by bleeding at the nofe, nor vomiting of blood, ufually owe their appearance to an hemorrhage, from fome branches of the mefenteni veffels. This difcharge is very often, in fome degree, critical, and contributes to the cure of the difeafe. *Sed et exiftit,* fays Duretus (n), *dyfenterio quæ confolatur et eft cri- tica ut fanguinea ; et quæ lienofis fupervenit critica eft : et quæ fenibus hæmorrhagiæ loco.* If any of our rea- ders can doubt of the identity of the ftools, alluded to in this part of our work, with the dyfentery here mentioned by Duretus, he will eafily be convinced by confulting the whole of the paffage.

An evacuation of blood, in this way, is, therefore, very often advantageous, and efpecially if it be mo- derate. But it is, fometimes, fo confiderable, by reducing the patient to extreme weaknefs, that the phyfician muft give him fpeedy, and fuitable help. I have, generally, found a plentiful ufe of oxycrat, a very ufeful remedy in thefe cafes. I dif-

---

(n) Anrot. in Holleruim de morb. interm. Cap. 43.

folve

folve about an ounce of fugar in every pint of the oxycrat, that he may be able to take fufficiently of the acid, without offending the palate, or ftomach of the patient. When Lommius fays, *Si ruptâ intus venâ aut adapertâ fanguis dejicitur, is ab inferioribus locis fere purus fertur, parum nigrefcens: a fuperioribus autem protinùs ater, ac liquidæ pici fimillimus, quotamen tincta lintea rubent: ut hâc notâ is quoque facilé diffidere ab atrâbile poffit* (o) he evidently fpeaks from obfervations, and every practitioner, who is attentive. tho' in only very limited practice, will be able to fatisfy himfelf of their truth.

§ CXCIII. (* 20.)

" In the beginning of May, 1770, I vifited a
" man, who, during five days, had felt all the
" fymptoms of inflammation of the breaft, a difeafe
" then prevalent, and which denoted itfelf by an
" acute fever, pain in the fide, fpitting of blood,
" and difficulty of breathing. In this patient, there
" came on a retention of urine, which proved a
" fpeedy, and compleat crifis to the difeafe. This
" retention of urine continued four days, and du-
' ring this time, we occafionally had recourfe to the
" catheter. At the end of that time, the flow of
" the urine was re-eftablifhed, but without any re-
" turn of the difeafe, which had been terminated by
" this fingular crifis."

(o) Obfer. Medic.

I copy

I copy this fact, verbatim, from my journal. It proves, that I have sufficient reason for asserting, that a retention of urine may serve as a crisis to an Acute Disease. I have, besides, several times seen a retention of urine, take place in the course of similar diseases, so that the patient has required the use of the catheter, and this, without any disagreeable event. Sometimes, however, I have seen it occur in cases that were truly mortal. To appreciate, therefore, the Prognostic, that such a symptom affords, we are not to consider it alone, but with all the other that accompany it, so that if the retention that happens in an Acute Disease, causes the more alarming symptoms to diminish, or disappear, we may conclude it to be critical. I have thought it the more necessary to give this remark, on the opinion we are to form of the retention of urine, in these cases, because, the celebrated Houlier assures exactly the contrary, and seems evidently to attribute, to the spurious ischuria, or to a suppression of urine, all the passages of Hippocrates, where he seems to give a favourable Prognostic from the ischuria : while he considers the true ischuria, or the retention of urine, that occurs in an acute fever, as being constantly a sign of excessive weakness, and approaching death (p).

§ CCX.   (* 21.)

I have really seen Acute Diseases, and particularly inflammations of the breast, terminate in this way:

(p) Comment. 1 Coac. v. lib. 1.

and

and thefe critical fweats, feem to be diftinguifhable from thofe, which are the effect of the exacerbation of the fever, by following clofe after the horripilatis, without that previous drynefs of the fkin, which, in the exacerbations, and paroxyfms, is accuftomed to interpofe between the fhivering, and the fweat. I think with Houllei (q), that Hippocrates alludes to this kind of fweat, in his *Prænot. Coac* where he fays, *febris ardens fuperveniente rigore folvitur.*

§ CCLXII. (*22)

That the reader may not be deceived in the application that is to be made of this Prognoftic, I think it right to make fome few obfervations on the difeafe, to which it relates, and of which we have no fufficiently exact account, either in ancient or modern books.

The difeafe, to which I give, fimply, the name of *rheumatifm*, is what phyficians, and others, often call *gouty rheumatifm.* It may be diftinguifhed into acute, and chronic. The former is accompanied with an acute fever, and the pains are much more violent, than thofe of the chronic rheumatifm.

The fever, that accompanies the acute rheumatifm, is ufually remittent, and its exacerbations give it the type of a quotidian.

(q) Com. 1. in lib. iv. Coac. Sect 22.

Violent

Violent pains in the moveable articulations, are the characteristics of this disease; these pains usually begin in the knees, and commonly continue there for a day or two. They then affect, successively, and, as it were, alternately, the different joints of all the limbs; sometimes one or two only, but more commonly, many of them at a time; and return again, at different times, to the parts they had before attacked, and quitted.

These pains are, sometimes, so excruciating, that the patients cry out through fear, on the least appearance of any thing being likely to touch, or hurt them. We are, likewise, obliged, for the same reason, in many of these cases, to keep off the bed clothes, and other covering, from the pained part. They are not always, however, in the same degree, but have their vicissitudes of increase, and remission, which correspond with the exacerbations of the fever. In general, they are attended with considerable swelling, and especially of the wrists and knees.

The acute rheumatism is of various duration. It is seldom terminated in less than fourteen or fifteen days, and sometimes it runs out to forty, and even sixty. In some cases, the fever, and the pains, cease at the same time; whereas, in others, the pains continue, even after the fever has disappeared, and torment the patient, tho' in a less degree, during many months. Now and then the disease gives rise to tophaceous concretion in the joints, which interrupt, and, sometimes, wholly prevent their motion. Sometimes too, it occasions a dropsy of the knee

Q q   joint,

joint. The swelling of the knee, when the disease is in a certain degree, commonly affords a sensible fluctuation, which is evidently from an accumulation of synovia, within the capcular ligament. In general, however, this is soon dissipated. But not so, when it continues for some time, or after the fever has disappeared, for in these cases, it is often very difficult, and even altogether impossible, to be obviated by remedies.

This disease occurs, neither in old age, nor in infancy. I have, indeed, tho' very rarely, seen it in subjects of twelve or thirteen years of age, but then it was of less violence, and duration, than it is in patients, who are past twenty.

When the disease has attained its acmé, it often affects, tho' in a slight way, the articulations of the vertebræ, and of the lower jaw: sometimes, too, it infests the lungs, (probably affecting the membranes, and ligaments belonging to the bronchial cartilages) and occasions pain in the breast, difficulty of breathing, cough, spitting of blood, and in a word, the symptoms of pleurisy, or peripneumony: now and then, in these cases, the pulse is unequal, and intermits. However dangerous the state of the patient may seem to be, in these occasions, we are not to despair of his recovery. Experience proves to us, that the matter of the disease, has a disposition to produce neither suppuration, nor gangrene; but, adhering to its character of mobility, soon quits the new seat it has chosen in the breast, and returns back to the limbs.

Left

Left to itself, or affifted only by regimen, there can be no doubt, but that nature will cure this difeafe, without the ufe of remedies. The means fhe employs here, are, as in the other Acute difeafes, fever, hemorrhage at the nofe, and evacuations by ftool, fweat, or urine. The phyfician imitates, and affifts nature, in thefe cafes, by moderating the fever, by venæfection, and folliciting, in due feafon, evacuations by ftools, and fweat. He may, likewife, be very ufeful on thefe occafions, by mitigating the pain, and inducing fleep by narcotic medicines. However refpectable the authority of Sydenhám may be, I venture, as many others have done, to differ from him here. I think that opiates may be ufeful in thefe cafes, when prefcribed by a prudent phyfician. They do not feem, as he afferts, to fix the difeafe, and render it more difficult of cure. The great difference we obferve in the duration and obftinacy of this difeafe, feems to depend more on its primitive character, and on the particular difpofition of the fubject, than on our method of treating it. When a man has been attacked with pleurify, it will, perhaps, return again a fecond or third time, in the courfe of his life, or it may happen, that he feels no more of it. It is the fame with the rheumatifm.

The chronic rheumatifm is, likewife, known by the pains, which fucceffively attack the moveable joints, and are ufually accompanied by fwelling of the parts. This difeafe, is very obftinate, and fometimes laft fix months, a year, and even a much longer time; now and then, it continues through life. It rarely, tho' it fometimes occurs, that it is fatal to

the

the patient. When this does happen, the patient is deprived, by the violence of the difeafe, of all motion, and is reduced to a moft emaciated ftate, by a flow fever, and by the influence of the rheumatifm on his breaft. It more commonly happens, however, that they become lame, by the tophaceous concretions, or by dropfy of one, or both knees. I have, likewife, feen the flexer mufcles of the fore arm, become fo hard and retracted, as to contribute to abolifh the motion of the elbow.

Young people are more fubject to chronic rheumatifm, than thofe in more advanced life. It is not feen, I believe, in old perfons, nor are thofe who are born of gouty parents, more liable to it, than others.

Sydenham feems to have written accurately from obfervation, when in defcribing the rheumatifm, he fays, " *Æger atroci dolore nunc in hoc, nunc in illo* " *artu infeftatur, in carpis, humeris, genubus præfer-* " *tìm, qui locum fubindè mutans, viciffim illos occu-* " *pat*' (r). Riverius, on the other hand, feems not to agree with obfervation, when he fays, " *non* " *folum articuli, fed etiam media inter articulos fpatia,* " *mufculi nimirùm, &c. rheumaticos affectus experien-* " *tur*' (s). And Hoffman ftill lefs, in the following expreffions ; " *in rheumatifmo mufculi cum* " *eorum membrana communi, et tendinibus, ubi offibus* " *inferuntur, gravi dolore et fpafmo hinc indè in artu-*

(r) De rheumatifmo.
(s) De rheumatifmo.

" *bus*

" *bus aliifque corporis regionibus afficiuntur*" (*t*). The moveable articulations, and efpecially, thofe of the limbs, are the true feat of this difeafe.

It has, indeed, this in common with the gout; but it differs from it, in fo many refpects, that it would be fuperfluous to remark here, with a number of authors, that they have done well to defcribe the rheumatifm a-part, and diftinguifh it from the *arthritis*, a name, applied now, only to the gout, but under which, the rheumatifm has, fometimes, been defcribed : witnefs the following paffage from Hippocrates, in his book, *De Affect.* where the acute rheumatifm is pretty exactly defcribed.
" *Arthritis morbus, cum detinet corporis articulos ig-*
" *nis et dolor invadit. Corripit etiam acuta, et in alium*
" *atque alium articulum dolores acutiores et leviores de-*
" *cumbunt. Hic morbus ex bile et pituitâ oritur . . . .*
" *et brevis quidem et acutus eft : fed minime lethalis.*
" *Junioribus que magis quàm fenioribus contingere*
" *folet. . . . . Podagra veró ejufmodi omnium qui*
" *circà articulos oriuntur (affectuum) violentiffimus*
" *quidem eft ac diuturnitiffimus*" (*u*).

§ CCLXVII.

(*t*) Tom. ii p. 317.
(*u*) The ancients, fays the learned Sir John Pringle, (in his Obf. on the Dif of an Army,) gave the name of *arthritis*, to the affection of all the joints, whether the pain arofe from rheumatifm, or gout. If not all, but fome particular joint fuffered, the diftemper was denominated from the part ; hence the terms *chiragra, podagra,* &c. Thefe pains differing from each other, they diftinguifhed them, according to the different humours, which they fuppofed to be the caufe of the difeafe. The word ρευματισμὸ, occurs, indeed, in Galen, but feemingly, only in
the

§ CCLXVII. (* 23.)

Petechiæ ufually appears, between the fourth, and feventh day of thefe fevers. They are of a red colour, varying however in the deepnefs of the tinge, and are as fmall as a pin's head. They feem to me to rife a little above the furface of the fkin, but they muft be nearly, and carefully examined, for us to obferve this. Thefe exanthemata, are, in general, diftinct; fometimes, however, feveral of them uniting, they form a large fpot. The eruption, in fome patients, is general, over the whole body; in others, it is confined to the back, or loins, or thighs. It is of a changeable nature, diminifh-ing, or increafing, or difappearing, and returning again feveral times during the courfe of the difeafe. It is pretty conftantly preceded, and accompanied by a troublefome cough, which has occafioned the difeafe, to be called by fome writers, catarrhal pe-techial fever. Fevers of this fort, are not always due to a manifeft corruption of the air. They often appear, without our being able to refer them to any known, and fenfible caufe. If my teftimony could add any weight to the opinion of the many cele-brated men, who have faid it before me, I would

---

the lax fenfe of *rheum*, or fluxion, and not to denominate any particular diftemper. Ballonius is the firft, who feems to have ufed the word *rheymatifm*, to denominate this inflammatory fpe-cies of arthritis, which he conceived to differ from either gout or catarrh; and we fee him beginning his treatife on the rheu-matifm, by calling it, *affectus pœne*, ανωγυς, *apud antiquos.*

add,

add, that experience clearly proves this eruption
to be due to the specific nature of the fever which
produces it, and not to any particular regimen.
Hitherto, in this country, I have seen fevers of
this kind, only in winter, or the beginning of
spring (x).

§ CCLXVIII.   (* 24.)

The purple spots do not rise above the surface of
the skin. They are usually circular, and about
as large as flea bites; from which they vary, however, in having no little point in the centre, as is
the case with flea bites. They likewise differ from
the latter in their colour. The purple spots being
commonly of a deeper, and sometimes wine colour,
approaching to violet. It would seem, as if authors
have, sometimes, confounded purple, with petechial
fevers; altho these two sorts of exanthemata, differ
very sensibly from each other; indeed, we sometimes, towards the close of fatal petechial fevers,
see an eruption of purple spots, which may then, at
the first glance, be clearly distinguished from the
petechiæ, that were there before them.

When a flea bite is of some standing, its disk is
effaced, and only the point, where the insect pene-
trated, remains tinged. When this point is recent,

(x) The reader will find the subject of *petechiæ*, very fully,
and ably treated, by Sr John Pringle, in his appendix, page
xcviii. et seq.

it

it is furrounded by a rofe coloured, circular difk,
almoft as large as a lentil. The true petechiæ, when
they are diftinct, refemble flea bites of fome ftand-
ing, while purple fpots, are more like recent flea
bites.

The miliary eruption is hitherto unknown in
Lower Languedoc, where I practice, and therefore,
being unable to fpeak of it from experience, I beg
leave to refer the reader to the many authors who
have written on the fubject (y).

§ CCLXXIV. (* 25)

I knew a perfon, who, every time fhe ate ftraw-
berries, felt, during the digeftion, a violent fhivering, which was fucceeded by fhivering, and a copious eruption on the fkin. Thefe fymptoms went
off after a few hours. I have likewife feen a ftudent
of phyfic, who, after drinking a little too much
Mufcadine wine, had an indigeftion with fhivering,
fever, and an eruption, which was fo general, over

(y) The beft authors feem now to be agreed, that the miliary eruption is, merely, the offspring of too hot a regimen,
that it is not occafioned by any fpecific matter, propagated by
contagion, and has, therefore, nothing critical in it, but may be
occafionally produced, under certain circumftances of fever,
heat, and fweating. Mr White, who has treated this fubject,
very much at large, in his ingenious Treatife on the Management of Pregnant and Lying-in-Women, has been at the pains
to collect together, in a note, the authors who have written on
the miliary fever; as follows: Sir David Hamilton, &c. &c —
See White's Treatife, page 32.

his

his face, as to disfigure him altogether, and to alarm himself, and his friends exceedingly. Before the next morning, it had totally disappeared. In France, we give the name of *porcelaine* to that sort of eruption, which resembles that, produced by the stinging nettle.

§ CCLXXV. (* 26)

In the remittent comatose fever, when it assumes the type of a double tertian, it would be only to prove our inexperience, to establish any hope of the happy event of the disease, on the observation of the lesser exacerbation, the symptoms of which, seem to be less alarming than those of the preceding fit. All the fevers, that have a similar course, and in the hemitritæa, the more violent exacerbations that occur every third day, are to be carefully compared with each other, that we may know whether they increase, or diminish.

§ CCCXXII. (* 27.)

Many authors have improperly considered this symptom as a particular kind of fever, which they have named *lypiria*. Experience, however, contradicts them, and proves, that this symptom is essential to no kind of fever, but that it pretty often comes on at the close of acute fevers, whether inflammatory or malignant, when they have a tendency to death.

R r   § CCCLXXXV.

§ CCCLXXXV. (* 28.)

Such was the practice of Sydenham, during the plague at London. Having observed, that the sweat was one of the means, nature took to terminate the disease favourably, he conceived, that it would be possible to bring on such a crisis, artificially; he began, therefore, by calming, by means of theriaca (z), the nausea, that tormented the patient; and he then caused him to be covered, and to drink plentifully of a sudorific decoction.

§ CCCCXV. (* 29.)

M. De Haen has written a dissertation on the critical days; and the conclusions he forms in it are quite contrary to my sentiments, on the subject. The celebrity of that writer, therefore, induces me to give here, my motives, for differing from so respectable an authority, in a matter of so much importance.

(z) The learned author, probably, had not Sydenham's works before him, when he wrote this note, but quoted him from memory.—Sydenham did not advise the theriaca, in these cases, to check the vomiting, but to act as a sudorific, when the patient was free from nausea.—" But," says he, " *if there* " *be a vomiting, as frequently happens in the plague—I forbear* " *sudorifics, till, by the weight of the bed clothes, a sweat begins* " *to appear, ... for then the vomiting ceases.*"

I have

I have already referred to the different paſſages, (*Hip.* 242, *& ſeq.*) in which Hippocrates contradicts himſelf, with reſpect to the critical days. Theſe oppoſite aſſertions being to be met with in works, that are equally high in the eſteem of phyſicians, and equally conſidered, as being the truly works of that celebrated man, we cannot but be at a loſs, how to determine, what was his true doctrine, on this head. Galen has endeavoured to reconcile theſe paſſages, or rather, to determine which of them ought to be preferred · and, according to him, the fourth, the ſeventh, the eleventh, the four-teenth, the ſeventeenth, and the twentieth, are to be conſidered as the principal days.

To M. De Haen, Galen's explanation is not ſuf-ficiently ſatisfactory. He aſcribes the contradic-tions that occur in the writings of Hippocrates, to the negligence, and inaccuracy of the copyiſts, who might eaſily give riſe to the miſtake, by ſubſtitu-ting one numerical letter for another (*a*). He therefore

---

(*a*) The reader, who has not the writings of M. De Haen, in his poſſeſſion, will not be diſpleaſed, to ſee here, the paſſages alluded to by the author. Græcis moris eſt numeros literis ut exponant . . . . . nunc ante inventam typographiam libri omnes ſtylo vel calamo exarabantur, quique ſcribendi arte vic-tum quæritærent, veloces eos in opere illo eſſe oportebat, nil committendis in eo erroribus facilius fuit. Potiſſimum ſi manu-ſcriptorum vetuſtas vietas literas contineret. Unde nam aliter manuſcriptorum compluuium varietas tum ſtupenda, tantaque contradictio nata ? Id quod eruditus *Foecius* toties acerbiſſimé

conqueſtus

therefore concludes, that if we had no other way to determine the difpute concerning critical days, than the reconciliation of thefe contradictory paffages, tho queftion would ever have remained in a ftate of uncertainty. But, fays he, we have two other means of deciding it, by confulting the obfervations of Hippocrates, and by our own experience. He, therefore, confulted the chemical obfervations of the divine old man, and from thence, was enabled to draw out the following table of critical days, in two hundred cafes.

---

conqueftus eft. Ita ut ad locum, de quo agitur, epidemicorum plurima exemplaria diffona invenerit : tribus antiquiffimis octavum diem reticentibus; duobus aliis decimum, ac vigefimum octavum; apponentibus vero, qui non in prioribus, diem vigefimum et vigefimum quartum. Iterum aliis exemplaribus expungentibus diem quadragefimum octavum, ejufque loco quadragefimum quartum laudantibus; aliis addentibus poft centefimum, vigefimum. Nofque hodie in Aph. iv 36. legimus 21 diem: Galenus legit 20, et veriffimé quidem; in omnibus vero Celfi exemplaribus 21 notatus fuerit.

Merito proinde concludimus notarios, five antigraphos, fimilitudine literarum, numeros defignantium, deceptos fuiffe, quod in victis manufcriptis facile; faepius ve eofdem numeros, quod feftinantibus folemne, omififfe. Adeo hoc Galeno perfuafum ut quod *Pythis* tertio *Epid.* non xi. fed x. die obiiffe legatur, librariorum erroriad fcribat. *Rat. Medend.* Tom. i. p. 20, *et feq.*

DAYS.

DAYS.	CRISES.
The third day afforded 7 crises,	3 good, 3 bad, 1 good, but uncertain as to the day.
The fourth -- -- 12	6 good, 6 bad.
The fifth -- -- 14	4 good, 5 with relapse, 4 bad, 1 fatal, but uncertain as to the day.
The fixth -- -- 25	13 fatal, 11 with violent relapse; 1 doubtful, whether it belongs to the 6th, or not, good, however.
The seventh -- 28	11 fatal, 8 complete, 9 uncertain, or with relapse.
The eighth -- -- 4	1 good, 2 fatal, 1 with relapse. It was the same with all the diseases of this constitution.

DAYS.

DAYS.		CRISES.

The ninth - - 6 $\begin{cases} 3 \text{ fatal,} \\ 1 \text{ with relapfe,} \\ 2 \text{ good.} \end{cases}$

The tenth - - 3 $\begin{cases} 2 \text{ bad,} \\ 1 \text{ with relapfe.} \end{cases}$

The eleventh - 9 $\begin{cases} 3 \text{ bad,} \\ 4 \text{ good,} \\ 2 \text{ either doubtful or with} \\ \quad \text{relapfe.} \end{cases}$

The twelfth - - 5 $\begin{cases} 2 \text{ fatal,} \\ 1 \text{ good,} \\ 2 \text{ imperfect.} \end{cases}$

The fourteenth 19 $\begin{cases} 3 \text{ bad,} \\ 15 \text{ good,} \\ 1 \text{ with relapfe.} \end{cases}$

The fifteenth - 2 $\begin{cases} 1 \text{ good,} \\ 1 \text{ bad.} \end{cases}$

The fixteenth - - 1 bad.

The feventeenth - 8 $\begin{cases} 6 \text{ good,} \\ 2 \text{ bad.} \end{cases}$

The eighteenth - 2 $\begin{cases} 1 \text{ good,} \\ 1 \text{ doubtful.} \end{cases}$

DAYS.		CRISES.

The nineteenth - -   1 good.

The twentieth - 16 $\begin{cases} \text{10 good,} \\ \text{1 imperfect,} \\ \text{5 bad.} \end{cases}$

The twenty-first -   1 bad.

The twenty-second   2 $\begin{cases} \text{1 good,} \\ \text{1 with relapse.} \end{cases}$

The twenty-third   1 $\begin{cases} \text{doubtful, whether it be-} \\ \text{longs to that day or} \\ \text{not.} \end{cases}$

The twenty-fourth   4 $\begin{cases} \text{2 bad,} \\ \text{1 good,} \\ \text{1 with relapse.} \end{cases}$

The twenty-fifth.   1 $\begin{cases} \text{bad, doubtful, however,} \\ \text{whether it belongs to} \\ \text{that day, or not.} \end{cases}$

The twenty-seventh   2 $\begin{cases} \text{1 good,} \\ \text{1 bad.} \end{cases}$

The twenty-ninth   1 $\begin{cases} \text{with relapse, untill the} \\ \text{40th day. It was the} \\ \text{same with all the dif-} \\ \text{eases of this constitu-} \\ \text{tion.} \end{cases}$

DAYS.

DAYS.		CRISES.
The thirty-fourth	2 {	1 good, 1 fatal.
The fortieth	12 {	8 good, 2 fatal, 2 doubtful, or with re- lapfe.
The fifty-firft - -		1 good.
The fixty-feventh -		1 bad.
The feventieth -	2 {	1 (perhaps) good, 1 bad.
The feventy-fifth -		1 good.
The eightieth -	4 {	3 good, 1 fatal.
The hundredth - -		1 good.
The hundred & twentieth		1 bad.

This is the table, M. De Haen has given to us, and this, as well as the conclufions he draws from it, I will beg leave to confider, with that freedom, which is fo effential to an enquiry after truth.

If

If that celebrated writer, will not allow us to attend to the contradictory passages we meet with in the dogmatical writings of Hippocrates, concerning the critical days, because the copyists may have given us one numerical letter for another; how happened it, that the same difficulty did not occur to him, in the clinical observations? It would seem, that if the copyists committed several mistakes in the transcribing of five or six passages, they would be equally liable to commit a greater number, in transcribing two hundred observations; and, therefore, having often written one day for another, no dependence can be had on these observations, to determine the doctrine of critical days. We must, therefore, admit all the contradictory passages on the critical days, that are to be met with in the writings of Hippocrates, and endeavour, with Galen, to conciliate them, or to select those which seem to claim the preference; or if we suppose them to have been wholly changed by the negligence of the copyists, we certainly should suppose this, as well of the clinical, as of the dogmatical writings, and ought, therefore, to give up all thoughts of deducing from them, the doctrine of critical days.

It would seem, altho' M. de Haen does not expresly say it, that he extracted these two hundred observations from the *epidemics* of Hippocrates. It is well known, how high the first and the third of these books stand in the estimation of the learned. In these are contained the histories of forty-two acute fevers. But the second, the fourth, and the sixth books of the epidemics, can, by no means be compared to the others. The best critics suppose them

S f

to be fpurious, or at leaft collected from fome fcat-
tered obfervations that might have been found a-
mongft the papers of Hippocrates. The fifth, and
the feventh, are more worthy of that great man, and
contain interefting obfervations. But a great many
of thofe contained in the fifth book, are repeated
verbatim in the feventh.

M. de Haen would, therefore, have done well
to have informed us, from what books of the epidemics, he derived the hundred and fifty terminations
of acute fevers, which he affociates and confounds
with the forty-two celebrated obfervations of the firft
and third books. We fhould then have been able
to have determined, with more precifion, what degree of confidence his table is entitled to. The
critical reader, who, from a defire to weigh, properly, both my arguments, and thofe of M. de
Haen, is induced to go through the fecond, and the
four laft books of the epidemics, will, with difficulty,
find a number of obfervations, fufficiently clear and
diftinct, to deferve to be confounded with the forty-
two cafes of the firft and third books, fo as to make
up the two hundred cafes, which according to M.
de Haen, are to eftablifh the doctrine of critical
days. He feems, himfelf, to have been aware of
this difficulty, in the following paffage: *Nemo
authoritatem hujus doctrinæ pondufque indé labefactori
autumet, quod ad eandem probandam non nulla funt
ex ejufmodi petita operibus quorum Hippocratis ne fint,
an aliorum, fit dubia fides.* He replies to it, however, by faying, that of the feventy books of differ-
tations which form the works of Hippocrates,
there are only twenty-four, confidered by our critics

as

as not belonging to him, but as having been collected from his papers, by his fons Theffalus and Draco, and his fon-in-law, Polybius ; and that Galen, Celfus, and the moft enlightened commentators of Hippocrates, confidered even thefe as very valuable. The reader will, with me, probably not be fatisfied with fo vague an anfwer. See what the learned Baron Haller fays, on the fecond and four laft books of the epidemics, in his edition of the *Principes Medicinæ*. See, likewife, the commentary of Galen on the fecond book of the epidemics.

But are the deductions M. de Haen infers from the above table peifectly exact? And fuppofing all the obfervations, on which it is founded, to be accurate and authentic, does it effectually prove the folidity, and utility of the doctrine of critical days? Thefe are queftions, that we will now endeavour to determine.

Every thing confidered, fays M. de Haen, the 24th aphorifm, of the 2d fection *(b)*, is that which agrees beft with the obfervations of Hippocrates, and which, of courfe, has been the leaft corrupted. According to thefe obfeivations, the third, fourth, fifth, feventh, ninth, eleventh, fourteenth, feven-

---

(b) Index feptimi quartus, fequentis feptimanæ octavum initium. Spectandus etiam eit undecimus, fiquidem is fecundæ feptimanæ quartus eit Ruifumque decimus feptimus fpectandus· is enim à quarto decimo quartus eft, fed ab undecimo, feptimus. *Aph.* 24 *Sect.* 11.

teenth,

teenth, twentieth, and fortieth, are the principal
critical days (*c.*)

These two assertions are, evidently, contradictory to each other. If the aphorism, quoted by M.
de Haen, is that, which agrees the best with the
observations, and has been the least changed,
the doctrine of Hippocrates, on the critical days,
such as Galen seems to have fixed it, (See § cccxci.)
is consistent with experience ; and if so, we ought
to erase from the number of these days, the third,
fifth, and ninth, neither of which, are mentioned in
this aphorism, or if these days are to be considered
as critical, we must allow, that the aphorism in
question, is one of those which have been the most
changed, whereas the 36th aphorism, of the 4th
section (*d*), would then seem to be more per-
fect.

Does that part of M. de Haen's table, which
relates to the eighth day, seem to differ sufficiently from that which relates to the ninth, to authorize
us to consider the latter only, as one of the principal critical days ; and to exclude the former ?

(*c*) Ex omnium autem recensione elucescit id, quod Aph.
2 —24. Omnium maximé cum observatis Hippocraticis con-
veniat, adeoque omnium minime corruptus fit. . . . . ,
Secundum hæc observata maxime critici sunt dies, 3, 4, 5, 7,
9, 11, 14, 17, 20, 40. *Rut. Mcæend. Tom.* 1.

(*d*) Sudores febricitantibus boni sunt et judicatorii.

Shall

Shall we simply give the name of critical days,
to those on which Acute Diseases the most commonly terminate, either well or ill ? Or taking this definition in good part, which deserve to be remarked
by the frequency, and solidity of favourable crises,
that take place on them? taking, as most people do,
the expression in the latter sense, it must be con-
fessed, that M. de Haen's table discomposes, and
contradicts, in a singular manner, the ideas we are
favoured with, of critical days, by all the writers
who are attached to the doctrine.

The seventh day, which has always been so famous
amongst the critical days, a day, that Galen compared to a benevolent prince, appears here, under
a very different aspect. Eleven deaths, to eight
complete crises, authorize us to consider it as a very
alarming day, on which nature seems rather to effect the destruction, than the recovery of the
sick.

The observations, which relate to the third fourth,
ninth and eleventh days, give rise to similar reflections.

According to the doctrine of Galen, and all his
followers, the fourth day, was in the opinion of
Hippocrates, the most remarkably critical. M.
de Haen's table, is, however, contradictory to this :
he represents the fifth, as being more favourable
than the fourth, because the latter had as many
deaths, as critical terminations in health, that happened on it ; whereas, of the same number of cases
on

on the fifth, there were a third, that ended in death ; a third, good ; and a third, incomplete.

The third, and the ninth days, which M. de Haen confiders as critical days, have been excluded from that rank, by almoft all the Hippocratic phyficians who have been attached to the doctrine of critical days.

If I likewife might be permitted to draw my confequences from a fimilar table, fuppofing it to be founded on obfervations, that are authentic, and fufficiently defcribed, I would fay, that it proves the 3, 4, 5, 6, 7, 11, 14, 17, and 20 days, to have been the moft common periods of the acute fevers, to which thefe obfervations refer. That the fourteenth day was, without contradiction, the moft favourable ; next to that, the twentieth ; and then the feventeenth : and, that there would only remain to inquire, whether the difeafes that were favourably terminated on thofe days, were fo by crifes which began and were ended on the fame day, or whether they did not terminate in the way of folution (e) ; and laftly, whether, when Hippocrates, fays of a difeafe, *judicatus eft*. he does not often allude to this mode of termination, and not always to a crifis properly fo called.

It would, likewife follow, from this table, that the feventh, and the eleventh, procured, indeed,

---

(e) See § cccccvi, ccccvii.

complete

complete crifes, as well as the third, fourth, and
fifth ; but, then the deaths on thofe days, are in fo
great a propoition, when compared with the terminations in recovery, that we cannot venture to confider them as favourable critical days. It would
therefore, be very imprudent to regulate in any degree, the Prognoftic and treatment of an Acute
Difeafe, on the confideiation of fuch or fuch
of thefe critical days, on which it would feem, it
ought to terminate, fince this confideration, is in no
way, capable of encouraging us, and becomes of no
weight, when compared with thofe we have mentioned, § cccxiv.

Might we not, likewife conclude, from this table,
that, in general, we have reafon to dread thofe acute
feveis, the alarming fymptoms of which appear fo
rapidly, as to difpofe them to terminate between the
fourth and feventh day; fince we find that thefe
four days afford, without comparifon, the greateft
number of deaths, and that the fevers, which run
on to the fourteenth, aie much lefs fatal. See
§ cccv.

We ought, likewife, to confider, how much any
data, that are founded on fuch tables, may be in-
fluenced by chance, and the vaiious combinations
of different cafes ; we fhould, likewife, carefully attend to the confequences to which thefe data may
give rife. Let us take, for inftance, the collection
of forty-two authentic obfervations, which are to be
found in the fiift and third books of the epidemics :
their terminations will be found to furnifh out the
following table.

In

In FORTY-TWO CASES.

DAYS.	CRISES.
The second day afforded a crisis,	{ 1 fatal. The ninth patient of the first book.
The third - - 1	{ 1 good. The eleventh patient, book 3, sect. 3.
The fourth - - 4	{ 3 fatal. The seventh patient, book 3, sect. 2. The fourth, and fifth, book 3, sect. 3. 1 good. The sixth patient, book 3, sect. 3.
The fifth - - 3	{ 1 good, somewhat imperfect. The seventh patient, book 1. 2 fatal. The eighth patient of book 1. The fourth of book 3. sect. 2.
The sixth - - 3	{ 1 good. The twelfth patient, book 3. sect. 3. 2 fatal. The first, and the eleventh patients of book 1.

DAYS.		CRISES.
The seventh	3	3 fatal. The eighth, tenth, and eleventh, of book 3, sect. 2.
The ninth	1	1 crisis, with relapse, the third patient of book 1.
The tenth	2	1 good, by expectoration. The first patient of book 3. 1 fatal. The third patient, book 3, sect. 3.
The eleventh	3	1 good. The fourteenth patient, of book 1. 2 fatal. The second and the twelfth patients of book 1.
The fourteenth	2	1 critical sweat, and vomiting, about the fourteenth day. The thirteenth patient of book 1. 1 fatal. The twelfth patient, book 3, sect. 2.

T t

DAYS.		CRISES.
The seventeenth -	3	1 good. The third patient of book 1. 2 fatal. The sixth, of book 3, sect. 2. and the fourteenth of book 3, sect. 3.
The twentieth -	2	1 good. The fifth patient, sect. 2. of book 3. 1 fatal. The fourth patient of book 1.
The twenty-fourth	2	1 good. The tenth patient, sect. 3. book 3. 1 fatal. The sixteenth patient, sect. 3. book 3.
The twenty-seventh	2	1 good. The seventh patient of book 3. sect. 3. 1 fatal. The second of book 3. sect. 1.
The thirty-fourth	2	1 good. The eighth patient, sect. 3. book 3. 1 fatal. The thirteenth of book 3. sect. 3.

DAYS.

DAYS.		CRISES.
Towards the fortieth 2	{	2 good. The tenth patient of book 1. and the third of book 3. fect. 1.
Towards the eightieth 3	{	2 good. The fifth patient of book 1. and the fixth. 1 fatal. The fecond patient of book 3. fect. 3.
Towards the 120th. 2	{	1 good. The ninth patient, fect. 3. book 3. 1 bad. The firft patient of book 3. fect, 3.

In all, forty-one cafes, twenty-three deaths.

The day, on which the feventh patient died, book 3. fect. 3. is not mentioned.

The above table proves, at firft fight, that if M. de Haen, had founded his data, wholly on thefe forty-two cafes, he would, neceffarily, have derived confequences, altogether repugnant to the doctrine of critical days. He would have faid, that the feventh is the moft unfavourable of all, becaufe it affords three deaths, and not one good crifis. The fixth, would have been lefs fatal, becaufe it gives only two fatal crifes, and one complete one. The

T t 2

fifth,

fifth, we see affording one favourble crifis, and three fatal ones. We find no termination on the ninth, and, therefore, this, and the fourteenth, which affords one death and one good crifis, would have been erafed from the lift of critical days. In fhort, the table would not have indicated one critical day.

If, therefore, chance was able to combine thefe forty-two cafes, we allude to, in fuch a manner, it will eafily be conceived, that the fame might have happened to two or three hundred, the refult of which would have been widely different from the conclufions of M. De Haen.

Thefe reflections are fufficient to prove, how far M. De Haen is from having demonftrated the utility, and truth of the doctrine of critical days. If any thing could induce us to adopt his opinion, it would be, his affurance, that his doctrines, on this fubject, agree with his experience. But my own interior conviction leads me in oppofition to the authority of that refpectable phyfician and to adhere to what I advanced in § ccccxiv. and which I believe to be agreeable to truth and nature.

§ CCCCXXXII. (˟ 30.)

Diffections prove, that in thefe fort of cafes, we fhould not be too hafty in concluding there to be metaftafis ; and that the inflammation, having quitted the lungs, is carried to the brain, or its meninges.

ninges. - After such symptoms, dissections often discover a very healthy brain, but a part of the lungs inflamed, and in a gangrenous state.

§ CCCCXLI.   (* 31.)

Spirationes quæ non nisi erectâ cervice ducuntur dirum hydropem faciunt. Hip. Coac. 424.

A mason, was in the twelfth day of a pleurisy. He seemed to be somewhat relieved, when he was affected with so violent a difficulty of breathing, that he was obliged to sit up in his bed, and even in this situation, he was able to breathe only with great difficulty. Two other physicians, and a very experienced surgeon, were called into consultation with me, and we all agreed, that the patient afforded, all the symptoms of an effusion into the cavity of the thorax. We were not permitted, however, to perform the operation for the empyema, and the patient died in less than four and twenty hours. After his death, I could only obtain leave to plunge a knife between the ribs, on the side in which we had reason to suspect an effusion, and there immediately flowed out a stream of a whitish serous fluid, that rose to the height of three or four inches.

This observation, together with those of the same kind, which we find in Morgagni (*f*), proves to

---

(*f*) De sedibus et causis morb. epistol. 21.   § XXXIV.

us,

us, the clear, and natural meaning of § cccxxiv, of the *Præn. Coac,* and which the beſt commentators have hitherto ſerved only to render more obſcure. The epithet σκληρος applied by Hippocrates to dropſy, may be underſtood in a figurative, as well as in its ſtrict ſenſe. Hippocrates uſed it in both theſe ways (*g*). Many authors, taking it in its ſtrict ſenſe, have rendered the Prognoſtic in this way : *orthopnæam facit hydrops durus*; others, inſtead of *durus*, have written *ſiccus.* I own, I have no conception of any diſeaſe that can be called a *hard dropſy* ; nor can I imagine, what affinity the difficulty of breathing can have with a dry dropſy, or tympanites. But taking the adjective σκληρος in a figurative ſenſe, and writing *orthopnæam facit dirus hydrops*, the meaning of the Prognoſtic will then appear to be very natural ; and this Prognoſtic occurring in that part of the *Coac.* where Hippocrates points out the ſigns peculiar to inflammations of the breaſt, we cannot help thinking, but that he derived it from obſervations ſimilar to ours. It is farther remarkable, that this Prognoſtic of the *Coac.* has an ultimate affinity with the fourteenth of the *Prænotiones*, which is conceived in the following terms : *Quod ſi dum morbus viget. ægrotus velit reſidere, hoc in omnibus acutis malum, in pulmoniis verò peſſimum.* The Prognoſtic of this ſymptom is ſaid to be the ſame in both works, but in the *Coac.* Hippocrates

(*g*) See the *æconomia Hippocratica* of Fœſius, at the ſame Greek word.

farther

farther infinuates that this fymptom depends on an effufion of ferum.

What then is to be the conduct of the phyfician, in thefe circumftances? Is he to abandon the patient to his fate, or will it be prudent to attempt to cure him by the operation for the empyema, or at leaft, by a puncture into the thorax? This is a nice and important queftion, to which we cannot reply, until we have particularly examined all the cafes, which having this difficulty of breathing as a common fymptom, differ. however, very effentially from one another, as to the fuccefs they would promife from fuch an operation.

It ought, in the firft place, to be remarked, that orthopnæa coming on in an inflammation of the breaft, gives room indeed to fufpect, tho' it does not prove there to be an effufion. This fymptom may be occafioned by inflammation of both lobes of the lungs, or by the polypous concretions in the heart, and great veffels, which fo often take place, towards the clofe of thofe difeafes. An example of this fort may be feen in Morgagni (h).

It will, therefore, not be fufficient, that orthopnæa comes on in a fimilar difeafe, to enable us to decide, whether the operation is to be performed or not; we muft carefully inquire, whether to this fymptom, there are not joined others which confirm

_____

(h) De fedib. et cauf. epift. 20. § xxiv.

the

the fufpicion of effufion. Thefe other corroborating
fymptoms, will be chiefly a fenfe of weight and inconvenience in the lower part of the breaft, together
with a fort of undulation within the breaft.

It feems, in fhort, to me, that the orthopnæa,
arifing from an effufion of ferum, comes on fuddenly, and fometimes in the very moment when the
patient gave hopes of a cure. But when it depends
on a violent inflammation and adhefion of the two
lobes of the lungs, it may be expected to come on
gradually. If it is occafioned, towards the clofe of
a fatal inflammation of the breaft, by polypous concretions in the heart, and great veffels, this caufe will
neceffarily be preceded and accompanied by all the
figns of a fudden and inevitable death.

Suppofing, that a careful examination of the patient confirms us in our opinion, that his orthopnæa
is occafioned by an effufion. ftill there remains to
be known whether this effufion has taken place in
both cavities, or on only one fide of the breaft.

If, during the courfe of a pleurify, we obferve
the figns of an effufion within the breaft, we have
reafon to prefume, that it is confined to the inflamed fide. If the patient defcribes the weight, and
inconvenience he complains of, as being confined to
this one fide, and is unable to lie, or even repofe
himfelf on the oppofite fide : if at the fame time,
we obferve that fide to be fenfibly larger, and more
expanded than the other, and on applying the hand
to it, we feel a fort of undulation, which is not to be
perceived in the oppofite fide ; we may then, from

all

all thefe figns, conclude the effufion to be only on that fide. It is in this cafe, therefore, that we may try the operation of the paracentefis of the thorax : efpecially if from the abfence of other alarming figns, we have reafon to confider this effufion, as the chief caufe that threatens the death of the patient.

In many cafes, without doubt, fuch an operation will be ineffectual, fometimes, becaufe the lungs, or the pleura, or mediaftinum, or pericardium, will have been fo affected by the difeafe, that death would have enfued, independent of the effufion. Sometimes too, it will be fruitlefs, becaufe the hydrothorax will, perhaps, be complicated with dropfy of the pericardium, the figns of which, are, as yet, too imperfectly known, to be able to determine us, with any degree of certainty, in thefe cafes.

The phyfician, therefore, who advifes the operation, has a right to expect, that in general, it will fail of fuccefs ; and he will do well, to inform the patients friends, that this laft refource fucceeds only with a very fmall proportion of the patients who are reduced to fo dangerous a ftate. But altho' not more than one in fifty may furvive it, yet ought we not to neglect to have recourfe to it.

§ CCCCXLIII. (ˣ 32.)

I am aware, that latterly, fome very refpectable writers, who have examined this matter, *ex profeffo,* have been led by their obfervations, and reflections,

U u

to affert, that this appearance of the blood, can afford no Prognoftic fign whatever. But I confefs, it is impoffible for me to be of their way of thinking, being certain, that the Prognoftics I have given, in § CCCCXLII. CCCCXLIII. are the refult of long experience, and a great number of obfervations.

§ CCCCLXIV. (* 33.)

A fervile fpirit has been no where fo predominant, as in phyfic. The very difeafe we are now fpeaking of, is a convincing proof of this truth. It was Galen, who afferted, that in pleurify, the pulfe is conftantly hard, and all later writers have fervilely copied him, by faying the fame thing, in contradiction, as it were, to the obfervations they had every day an opportunity of making. There are pleurifies, in which the pulfe, from the very attack, fo far from being hard, is foft, fmall, and weak. This happens in the malignant pleurify. In inflammatory pleurify, the pulfe is fometimes hard, fometimes foft, and open; in certain cafes, very fmall; in others very much expanded. In a word, the pulfe is neither conftantly the fame, in all pleurifies, nor in any one, from the beginning to the end. It is wrong, therefore, to introduce hardnefs of the pulfe, into the definition of the difeafe.

§ CCCCLXVI. (` 34)

This, or I am deceived, is one of thofe cafes (fo frequent in phyfic) where our reafon muft fubmit

mit to obfervation. I have, indeed often feen, that inflammations of the breaft, which began with obftinate vomiting, were liable to exhibit, in their courfe, a purulent expectoration. But how are we to explain this? is a queftion, I will not attempt to anfwer.

§ CCCCLXLV. (* 35.)

It is neceffary to caution the inexperienced practitioner, againft an error of Prognoftic, which I have often feen committed. A pleurify, or peripneumony being followed by a remittent or intermittent fever (at leaft, in appearance) that affumes the type of a tertian or quotidian; and each paroxyfm beginning with a fhivering fimilar to that which occurs in a true intermittent; I have feen the phyfician confider and treat it as an intermittent. A more inftructed practitioner, however, will not eafily fufpect, that a fever of this kind can eafily fucceed a pleurify or peripneumony; but comparing the progrefs of this fever, with all the other fymptoms of the difeafe, he will difcover it to be a fuppurative fever.

§ CCCCLXXXIX. (* 36.)

To confirm what I advance in this paragraph, I will tranfcribe a cafe, written by me, in 1752. I give it as it occurs in my collection. " Hunc mor-

bum

" bum, (pulmonis tuberculum (*i*), vidi apud Ar-
" naud cui, cum jamdiù tuffiret ac dolorem per-
" fentifceret in pectore, in cervicis parte porticâ,
" imò et fecundùm brachia, itâ ut alterutrum attol-
" lere fine dolore non poffet, obfervata eft inter fe-
" cundam et tertiam coftas lateris dextri pulfatio
" valdè manifefta, quæ me ipfum et alios aneuryf-
" matis opinione fefellit. Tuberculum maturatum
" ruptumque (ut pus per expectorationem ingenti
" copiâ prodiret) aneuryfmatis fpeciem penitus fuf-
" tulit. Similis tumor aneuryfmatis opinione Bal-
" lonium decepit. *Epid. lib.* 2."

§ DXVI.　(ᵃ 37)

It is this fort of abfcefs, that is defcribed by Hippocrates (*k*), under the name of tubercle of the
lungs. " Tuberculum in pulmone fit hoc modo.
" Cum pituita aut bilis coacta putrefcit : Et quam-
" diu quidem adhuc crudius fuerit, dolorem exilem
" ac tuffim ficcam inducit. Poftquam autem matu-
" ratum fuerit, dolor et ante et retrò acutus fit, et
" calores corripiunt ac tuffis vehemens. Et fi
" quidem quàm citiffimè maturuerit et eruperit, et
" pus fursùm vertatur, ac totum expuatur, et ventri-

(*i*) There is queftion, in this part of my collection, of the
tubercle of the lungs, defcribed by *Hippocrates de morb.* *Lib.* 1.
The reader will fee what I fay of it in § DXV. *et feq.*

(*k*) *De morb.* *Lib.* 1. See likewife, *Lommii.* *Obf. Med.* p.
120, and the preceding note.

" culus

" culus in quo fuerat pus, contrahatur ac reficcetur,
" penitus fanúfevadet, &c." This tubercle of the
ancients, was therefore, very different from that to
which the moderns have given the fame name.
That of the ancients was properly an abfcefs;
whereas, the moderns underftand by tubercles,
hard glandular fwellings, which forming in the lungs
excite cough and fever, and at length degenerating
to ulcers *mali moris*, bring on confumption,

§ DXXVI. (* 38.)

All that I fay here, on the fubject of lymphatic
vomica, (§ cccxxi, et feq.) is founded on obfervation. I have feen every thing that I mention in
§ DXXII, et feq. to DXXV. The conjecture in
§ DXXVI. is likewife founded on obfervation. I was
called in the night, to fee a lady aged thirty years,
who fix months before had brought up a lymphatic
vomica, and had efcaped the phthifis with which
fhe was threatened. She died, fuffocated before I
could get to her. I conjectured that a new vomica
fimilar to the former one, and which fhe could not
bring up, had occafioned her death ; but I could
only conjecture, as the friends would not permit me
to open the body.

§ DXXXIX. (* 39)

When a patient dies from fuch an hemorrhage, it is
ufually the affair of a few minutes only; blood in
fuch a cafe, is thrown up in great profufion, either
from

from the rupture of some aneurism, which discharges itself into the bronchiæ, or because an ulcer of the lungs has destroyed the coats of some of the great vessels. In a great number of consumptive patients, we see some few who die in this way. But so long as the expectoration of blood, is no more than a simple hemopthysis, that is, so long as the patient spits up blood only by coughing, we have no reason to fear a similar event. It is the more necessary to caution the young physician on this head, as the desire of stopping the discharge too suddenly, has often led to great errors in the treatment of this delicate disease.

§ DLII. (* 40.)

It is essential, to be acquainted with the symptoms that are the usual forerunners of apoplexy, because it may be sometimes in our power to correct the disposition to it, by exercise, regimen, &c: whereas, if it once takes place, it either proves immediately fatal, or leaves behind it, infirmities, which often continue during life. Amongst the signs that denote the predisposition to apoplexy, we may include fixed and obstinate pains in some part of the head, as a leading sign. We frequently meet with paralytic patients, who complain of having felt this during a month or two previous to their first attack of apoplexy, or hemiplegia.

§ DLVI.

§ DLVI.   (* 41.)

The definitions of apoplexy we fometimes hear in the fchools, and which we meet with in a variety of authors, are liable to lead the young phyfician into the moft ferious errors. If we define to him apoplexy, as being a fudden privation of all feeling, and voluntary motion; with ftertor: we do not give him a definition which is general enough to include all the cafes which the experienced practitioner will difcover to be apoplectic. We only define to him the apoplexy, which is violent, and fatal. We fhould, therefore, inform him, that this difeafe will occafionally vary much as to its degree of violence : that fometimes it deftroys the patient inftantaneoufly, and at others, agrees with the definition, we have juft been criticizing, and then may be confidered as the violent and fatal apoplexy of Hippocrates ; that in other cafes the lofs of fenfibility, and motion, is far from being fudden, but takes place by degrees. In fhort, that there are apoplexies in which the refpiration is without ftertor, and in which the patient preferves the power of fwallowing ; more or lefs of motion and fenfibility, when pricked or pinched ; and on which, when tormented to a certain degree, he opens his eyes, and even pronounces fome few words.

THE END,

INDEX.

A

B.

Empyema,

X x z   Hemorrhages

Page:

Paralytic

T.

V.

W.

The EDITOR, *having been at too great a Distance from the Press, whilst the Work was printing, to be able to correct the Sheets himself, begs the Reader to excuse the following* ERRATA.

Page vi of the Preface, second Line from the Bottom, *for* to thofe, *read* of thofe.
    xv *for* extends, *read* extend.
    171 *for* Empiema, *read* Empyema.
    193 *for* apthalmia, *read* opthalmia.
    274 *for* bube, *read* bubo.
    288 *for* fuint, *read* fiunt.
    293 *for* Mefenteri, *read* Mefenteric.
       for morb. interm. *read* morb. intern?
    294 *for* tineta, *read* tinta.
    295 *for* other, *read* others.
       for affures, *read* afferts.
    296 *for* horripilatis, *read* horripilatio.
    297 *for* concretion, *read* concretions.
    298 *for* capcular, *read* capfular.
    300 *for* flexer, *read* flexor.
       for experientur, *read* experiuntur.
    301 place the comma after *detinet,* inftead of *morbus.*
    302 *for* appears, *read* appear.
    305 *for* All the fevers, *read* In all the fevers.
    307 *for* truly, *read* true.
    308 *for* erroriad fcribat, *read* errori adfcribat.
       for chemieal, *read* clinical.